Raw Vegan Recipe Fun for Families

115 Easy Recipes and Health Tips for Energetic Living

by

Karen Ranzi, M.A.

DISCLAIMER

The information contained herein is not intended as a diagnosis, cure or treatment for any disease or ailment. Because an initial cleansing and detoxification reaction can often occur as a result of a simpler and cleaner diet, parents and all readers are advised to properly educate themselves and seek advice from a qualified health professional when needed. The author does not accept any liability or responsibility for any loss, injury, or damage, or any adverse consequences that may be encountered from following any information in this book.

Editor: Professor Joel Brody
Proofreading: Brian Rossiter of Fruit-Powered.com
Cover and book design: Anna Chmielewska of SweetVeganNature.com and annacdesign.com.
Food photos taken by Karen Ranzi; Anna Chmielewska; Ramapo College interns Kelsey Higgins and Jacqueline Todaro.
Cover family photo and Karen's back cover photo: Dorothy Salvatori of DorothySalvatori.com.
Cover family photo (from the left): Margrieta (Grieta) Lasmane (wife), Mikus Lasmanis (husband), Jasmina Lasmane (daughter), Gundars Mikos Lasmanis (son).
Photo of Karen Ranzi on About the Author page: Julia Lucas of JuliaLucas.com
Photo of Karen and Gabriela Ranzi at the Raw Living Expo: Michele Marie Jeppson of SuperRawLife.com

ISBN-13: 978-1492748229
Published in The United States of America.

Acknowledgements

I would like to offer special thanks to my editor, Joel Brody, book designer, Anna Chmielewska, and proofreader, Brian Rossiter. I'm also grateful to the raw vegan chefs who have contributed healthful recipes to Raw Vegan Recipe Fun for Families.

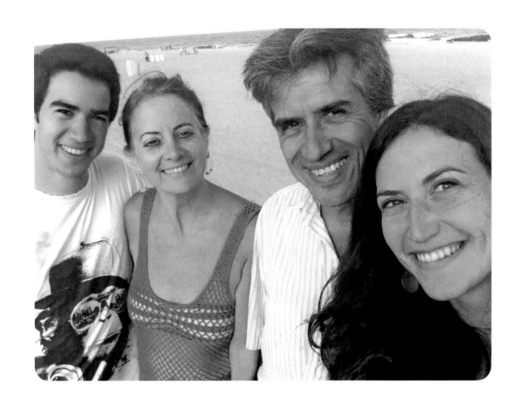

I dedicate this book to my husband, Harvey, and my wonderful children, Gabriela and Marco, who have taught me so much about living life, laughing, loving, and learning.

FOREWORD

In one way, the United States owes its birth to John Montagu, the Fourth Earl of Sandwich, but will the nation's continued health be imperiled by his invention? During the years of the American Revolution, John Montagu was the First Lord of the British Admiralty. He was too busy with his gambling, deflowering young maidens, and worrying about a naval war with France, so he simply didn't send enough troop ships to the colonies for England to win the war. Ironically, this is not his claim to fame. It's the following: One day in 1762, while playing cards at his posh London club for 24 hours straight, his servant came to inform him that the dining room would soon close. If the Earl wanted dinner, he would have to get up from the gambling table and go to the dining room. Instead, he chose not to move and asked his servant to bring him a slice of roast beef between two pieces of bread. He needed the bread to absorb the grease, so he could play cards. When the other gamblers saw what Sandwich was eating, they wanted it, too, and ordered their servants, "Get me what Sandwich is eating!" John Montagu, the Fourth Earl of Sandwich, unwittingly invented fast food. Although he unintentionally helped give the U.S. its nationhood, will his invention eventually destroy it internally with current medical costs and ever-increasing obesity?

I begin this preface to Karen Ranzi's book, *Raw Vegan Recipe Fun for Families,* with this historical event. Sandwich was thinking only of the expediency of the moment, his hunger during a 24 hour gambling binge, and not to have greasy fingers. He wasn't thinking of the digestibility of his invention. His fellow gamblers were attracted by the novelty—something new to eat. Who in the world would think of digestion when hungry? Karen Ranzi does with the recipes to follow. It's simply not enough for a recipe to be a taste and texture sensation. It must prove healthful in the long run.

A wonderful quality kicks in when we eat only one food at a time, the way all the animals in nature do. Animals in nature always eat mono meals. Lions get their meat, and seals get their fish, but never with bread, rice, pasta or potatoes. Yet recipe books abound mostly with hard-to-digest protein and starch combinations. A new restaurant was positively reviewed on TV for its innovative pasta dish with a mustard and pastrami sauce. People will try it, unaware of what it takes to digest something like that. As humans, we always want to do it better, improve on what exists and, even better, to invent something new and novel. We are forever building taller towers, more luxurious homes, fancier restaurants, and even last year's stiletto heels are not high enough for this year's fashionista.

Yet, when it comes to food, squirrels and sheep display more energy and health with their raw vegan mono meals than we do with our complicated combined fare. The wonderful quality of eating only one food at a time becomes apparent when one gets tired of eating that food—at first, amazingly delicious, but as we keep eating, it's just good and, finally, boring. Only then do we stop. But when foods are combined in recipes, all this changes.

Karen Ranzi's *Raw Vegan Recipe Fun for Families* contains simple transitional raw vegan recipes nearly all of which respect the requirements of food combining for easy and ideal digestion. Although recipes in general are never ideal, we have gotten used to eating for fun, parties, holiday gatherings, for which we want to heighten our experience and make it more memorable, more special. I remember how my uncle used to suffer every year after overeating at his office Christmas party. He was annually out of commission for 48 hours. His stomach rebelled. Why, I asked, did he have to go through this pain every year? Couldn't he remember his bitter experience from the previous year?

The recipes to follow will not upset the most sensitive stomach. They are designed to be a bridge from the cooked recipe world to the blissful, pain free raw vegan lifestyle, until the time when we'll enjoy one food at a time so much that recipes will no longer be of interest, and mono meals will be preferred to combinations. Then, to paraphrase the old song, *Life Will Really Be a Bowl of Cherries*.

In the meantime, I wish you the simplicity of health and happiness with Karen's delectable recipes.

—*Joel Brody, longtime raw vegan, and editor of Raw Vegan Recipe Fun for Families, Creating Healthy Children, and other books and articles on the raw vegan lifestyle.*

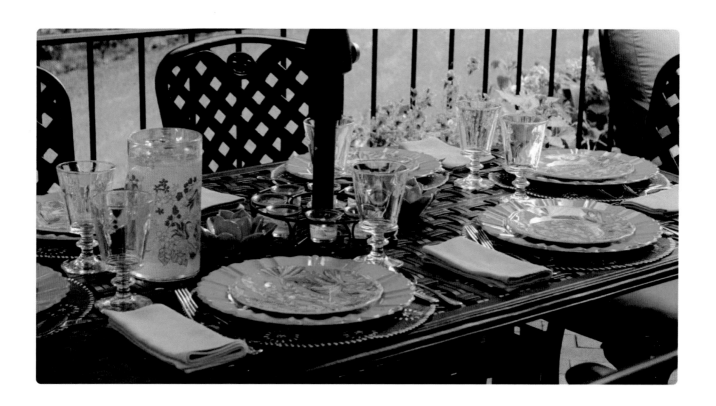

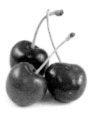

TABLE OF CONTENTS

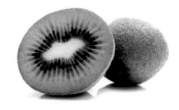

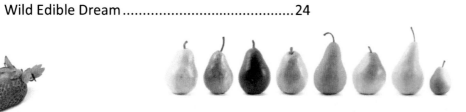

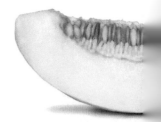

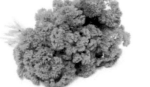

INTRODUCTION

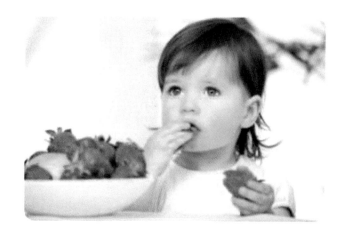

My name is Karen Ranzi. I'm passionate about helping families to achieve health and wellness in a distraught world, full of misinformation. I'm the author of a comprehensive book on raising healthy children from pre-conception to pregnancy to infancy to young children to older children to teenagers, *Creating Healthy Children: Through Attachment Parenting and Raw Foods.*

My website, SuperHealthyChildren.com, contains articles, recipes and information on raising truly healthy children through fresh plant nutrition. I also offer many YouTube videos on raising healthy families:

www.YouTube.com/superhealthychildren.

The classes and programs I offer include: Raw Food Private and Group Coaching, The Raw Food Challenge and Raw Food Fun for Families.

Since 1994, I have been living the raw food lifestyle. I embraced it following my son's healing from asthma, multiple food allergies and chronic ear infections on raw vegan foods. My paternal grandmother had turned to a high raw vegan lifestyle to heal her asthma and emphysema in the early 1920s, and I grew up hearing her story.

I've received many requests for a book that includes an abundance of simple raw food recipes that work for families on a daily basis. Much of our food should be eaten naturally as found in a garden, without the use of recipes, but the recipes in this book serve to begin increasing fresh plant foods for a more healthful lifestyle. Many families have asked me for my favorite easy healthful recipes. Most of the recipes are my own creations, and others come from raw food chef friends whose work in the raw food community I admire especially because their ingredients are pure and provide nutrients instead of anti-nutrients. I'm also providing helpful articles here that focus on nourishing our families to the fullest.

It's my sincere wish that these transitional recipes will bring you and your family abundant health and well-being. To receive ongoing family health tips, simple raw food recipes and a variety of articles, please sign up for my free monthly newsletter at

SuperHealthyChildren.com.

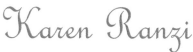

ABOUT THE AUTHOR

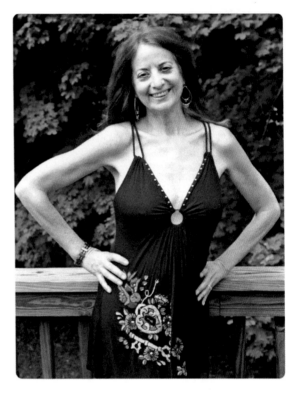

*A*uthor, speaker, speech therapist, and raw food consultant and chef, Karen Ranzi, M.A. authored and published her groundbreaking book, *Creating Healthy Children: Through Attachment Parenting and Raw Foods* in 2010. This latest book is all recipes and articles about healthy living titled *Raw Vegan Recipe Fun for Families*. Karen has been following a raw vegan lifestyle since 1994.

Karen travels throughout the United States and abroad delivering her impassioned message about raising healthy families. She has presented for universities, schools, health festivals and expos, health institutes and associations. In June 2012, Karen was the keynote speaker at the "Health Congress 'Flowers of Life,'" south of Moscow, organized by the Russian Association of The Raw Food Movement and Naturopathy.

Karen received enthusiastic audiences during her health and wellness workshops at the University of South Carolina, Penn State University, Lesley University and Ramapo College. She is a writer for Get Fresh! Magazine, VegWorld Magazine, Vibrance Magazine, Super Raw Life Magazine and Eternity Watch Magazine. Karen is Health Expert Advisor for http://SAFbaby.com.

Karen has been interviewed by Steven Prussack, host of *Raw Vegan Radio*, on "Interviews with the Raw Vegan Masters" and "RAWpalooza" and has been a featured guest on numerous TV and radio talk shows, including segments on Dr. Gary Null's *Progressive Radio Network* and *Living Consciously* with host Monty Taylor. Karen was also a featured guest on *The Conscious Foods Summit* and Matthew Monarch's *Conscious Parenting Summit*. Karen spoke for an audience of 250 chemists at the February 2012 Symposium of The New York Society of Cosmetic Chemists. Her topic focused on "Nutrition for Beauty and Health of the Skin: How Early Feeding Habits Affect the Skin in Later Years." In June 2012, Karen was a featured speaker covering "Beauty and Health of the Skin" at the New York Health and Beauty Expo at the Jacob Javits Center in New York City. More recently, Karen was interviewed on "Creating Healthy Children" and "Eating to Avoid the 'A' Disorders" on the *Living Healthy Show*, showing on 14 cable television channels and Peg Media. In November 2012, Karen was interviewed by Mitchell Rabin, host of *A Better World TV and Radio*. She was interviewed in May 2013 by Victoria Moran on *Main Street Vegan Radio*. Karen was nominated "Green Housewife 2012 to 2013" by Bergen Health & Life Magazine. In June 2013, Karen was the featured guest on Dr. Michael Finkelstein's radio program *The Skillful Living Room*, with a listener audience of 600,000.

On May 28, 2012, Karen Ranzi talked as author expert on "Attachment Parenting" with New York

Radio Host Mark Riley on WWRL 1600 AM, following the overwhelming national outcry to the sensational May 21st, 2012 Time Magazine cover, which showed a three year old boy breastfeeding.

In addition to her work in nutrition, Karen holds a Masters degree in speech pathology from New York University and is a speech therapist working with children of all ages since 1977, specializing with autistic children since January 2002. She incorporates nutrition therapy into her work with children on the autism spectrum and has observed impressive progress in their communication skills and their increased ability to focus and learn.

Every June, Karen supervises twenty speech pathology graduate students from northeastern universities as they work with autistic children at Camp Kaleidoscope of Vermont, a unique camp program for autistic children and their families. Karen increases her students' awareness of the impact of whole food nutrition on the children's health and wellbeing, which includes the benefits of a gluten free/ dairy free lifestyle, eliminating processed foods and increasing the amount of fresh raw plant foods.

Karen is a pioneer presenter for The Woodstock Fruit Festival since 2011, an event which occurs annually in August.

In 1994, Karen discovered the natural path that enabled her son to heal from asthma, chronic ear infections and multiple food allergies. By means of her education, life-changing personal experiences and sincere desire to share her message, Karen has been able to guide thousands of individuals and families toward developing excellent health. For more information, visit us at:

♡ SuperHealthyChildren.com

 facebook.com/CreatingHealthyChildren

 YouTube.com/SuperHealthyChildren

To set up a consultation or class with Karen, or to engage her as a speaker for your group, contact Karen at karen@superhealthychildren.com

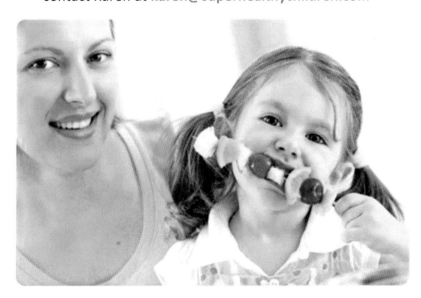

Articles and Health Tips for Families

Before immersing yourself into recipe-making fun, please enjoy understanding the foundation of the raw vegan lifestyle with the following articles.

Learn about the benefits of raw food for families, how to live most healthfully through simplicity, the importance of eating organic foods, and the most useful appliances for the raw vegan kitchen.

Benefits of The Raw Food Lifestyle for Families

There is abundant research showing the benefits of nutrient-dense fruits and vegetables. In 2007, the journal *Pediatrics* indicated how important it is for mothers to consume fruits and vegetables during pregnancy, and that these foods enter the amniotic fluid to create a child who will continue to love fruits and vegetables. The same happens with mother's milk. The fruits and vegetables from which mother makes her milk are delivered to the baby, who in turn will love these water-rich healthful foods. It is a much more daunting task to help children love these natural tastes when they have grown up eating the conventional foods, usually containing a high volume of animal flesh and animal products, processed and refined packaged foods, tragically devoid of nutrient-dense fruits and vegetables. To find a more detailed analysis of the nutrients in fruits and vegetables, see my first book, *Creating Healthy Children.*

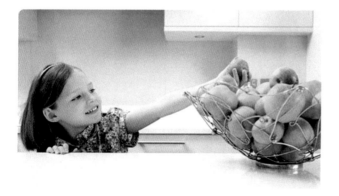

The following pages contain simple recipes for a healthy daily raw food lifestyle. Some think they can't do raw foods because it's too complicated, but the most healthful way to eat raw foods is to do so most simply. It's the quickest fast food there is! Grab a couple apples! Prepare simple green smoothies and green juices. It need not be labor intensive.

What is the reasoning for eating raw living plant foods? First, they are water-rich. Each fruit and vegetable contains all the water of that plant. Watermelon, for example, is 90% water. This is not like tap or spring water. It is the perfect water, filtered through the roots and branches of plants. Our bodies are reported to be approximately 72% water, so we need to constantly replenish that water. Most Americans eat only 5 to 10% water-rich fresh foods. Water is lost through the kidneys, bowels, lungs and skin, and the lost water must be continually replenished. This was one of the first benefits I observed on raw foods—the water-rich food I was eating would go in and come out very quickly. I noticed at certain times, especially in summer, when I was getting so much water from ripe melons, lots of delicious locally grown cucumbers and tomatoes and other fresh summer fruits, blended green soups, smoothies and green juices, I had absolutely no desire for additional water, as I was already receiving the right amount.

Our blood must have a slightly alkaline pH, but cooked foods, with the exception of lightly steamed vegetables or vegetable broths, are acid-forming. Foods are either acid-forming (acidifying) or alkaline-forming (alkalinizing). Acid fruits, such as oranges, even though acidic, leave an alkaline ash once metabolized by the cells. When oranges are exposed to high temperatures, such as in pasteurized orange juice, they lose their ability to form an alkaline ash, and remain acidic. We can only handle small amounts of acid-forming foods that acidify the body fluids. Dairy foods are high in sulfur and phosphorous, making them acid-forming. Dairy, grains (except millet), meat, refined sugars and nuts are high in the minerals that cause acidity. When the body is stressed from too much acid-forming food, it resorts to leaching alkalizing elements such as calcium from the bones and teeth to maintain the blood's correct level of alkalinity.

A most important reason to eat fresh plant foods is for their nutrient density. Studies report that cooking and processing foods cause the loss of many nutrients, especially Vitamin C, folate and Vitamin B1. When synthetic forms of these nutrients are added back to processed foods, they are not absorbed, and in the case of Vitamin E, the synthetic form does go to the receptor sites, only to block the absorption of the natural form. All cooked foods will lose some of their nutrient density, but some are clearly less harmful than others. Lightly steamed vegetables and whole grains such as millet, an alkaline grain, are some of the more healthful cooked foods.

Some of the many advantages your children will experience after significantly increasing their intake of fresh, unprocessed fruits and vegetables: absence of eye, ear, nose, throat or sinus infections; increased energy and attention spans; enhanced ability to process information; a heightened sense of ease, comfort, harmony and perception; less hyperactivity; strengthened immune systems; enhanced athletic capability; increased brainpower and intellectual curiosity; emotional poise; a greater range of expressivity; and improved sleep.

▲ ▽ ▲

The Raw Vegan Lifestyle Can Be Hazardous, If Not Lived Simply

Unfortunately, many new to the raw vegan lifestyle follow it haphazardly, eating a high volume of nuts and/or seeds, without realizing the amount of plant fat they are ingesting. In addition, dehydrating much of their food depletes the water content our bodies need. Not eating enough mineral-rich leafy green vegetables can compromise bone and dental health.

I encourage my audiences and readers to eat raw vegan foods because of their healing and health-promoting benefits and because they don't cause harm to animals or the environment. Indeed, they are nature's foods for us.

Just because a packaged food is labeled "raw" doesn't mean it is healthful or even raw. For example, agave nectar is no better than high fructose corn syrup. It's highly processed and nowhere near its natural state. Furthermore, it's not raw, just as cashews labeled raw are not raw. Moreover, health seekers avoid cashews due to their excessive amounts of Omega-6 compared with Omega-3 and because of the chemical process used to remove the shells. The majority of your foods ideally should be fresh and unpackaged. The food should not be heated above 118 degrees, the temperature at which nutrients begin to be depleted. Dehydrated food depletes water from foods. Maple syrup, another concentrated sweetener used in some raw food recipes, is not raw. The boiling down process creates the intense sweetness.

Many ingredients in raw gourmet cuisine are not at all healthful. For example, Nama Shoyu and Braggs Liquid Aminos are highly processed and contain excesses of sodium. In this book, you will not find these added to recipes to appease addictive tastes. I also recommend not adding table salt to recipes. I don't include any in my recipes for the following reason:

Salt, because of its toxicity, must be diluted in water in the cells, resulting in water retention. With time, the waterlogged cells begin to droop due to years of salt consumption, their consequent water retention and gravity. While adding salt enables the retention of the familiar tastes of cooked fare, once we're liberated from this extremely salty taste, we can move forward with greater freedom, energy and flexibility.

Did you know ...

Raw leafy green vegetables contain adequate amounts of organic mineral salts, supplying our ideal mineral requirements with excellent flavor.

Raw cacao, or chocolate, is a very stimulating substance containing *theobromine*, which has negative side effects. Every time I've had even a small amount, I was unable to sleep that night. We can get our magnesium needs met very well through green leafy vegetables and other plants, without resorting to super stimulating chocolate.

Vinegars, including balsamic vinegar and apple cider vinegar, are acids. My kids used to love combining vinegar with baking soda to create an explosion. That's exactly what will happen in your stomach. Oils are processed, fractionated and are 100% fat. Even a little equals a lot of fat. It's best to get our caloric needs met from fruits and smaller amounts of avocados, nuts and seeds (see the article *All about Nuts*, page 82). Kids, of course, will require more of the overt fat sources during times of increased physical activity and growth spurts. We must make these foods available and let our children listen to their needs for the more overt fat sources.

Some of the following recipes contain nuts, seeds and avocados. There is no added oil in any of the recipes. Pâtés, and other recipes containing more nuts and seeds, should be eaten as one or two scoops on a large high-mineral salad of leafy green vegetables, such as Romaine lettuce, spinach, arugula and other nutrient-dense fresh plant foods.

The recipes are designed for those transitioning to a high raw or totally raw vegan lifestyle desiring quick, easy, and tasty recipes. Not all the recipes reflect proper food combining, which I recommend on a daily basis for ease of digestion, particularly for adults. For that reason, I'm including a *Food-Combining Chart* (see page 72). As one's palate becomes acclimated to these more healthful natural foods, recipes will be needed less and less, and you will naturally get used to combining foods correctly.

Eating Organic

It's important for individual and family health to buy organic food. In 2013, 10% of the U.S. population is buying organic food.

In conventionally grown foods, many pesticides are taken up internally in the plant. Pesticides can cause adverse effects from cancer to nervous system damage and reproductive problems. Many pesticides mimic estrogen and become endocrine disruptors that affect hormone balance and have been associated with breast and prostrate cancer, deformities of the reproductive organs, fertility problems, altered fetal and child development, learning disorders and more. Of course, children are more vulnerable to the damaging effects of pesticides than adults.

Conventional farming contributes toxins in the air, water and earth. Because we know pesticides contaminate many fruits and vegetables, you should always choose organic if possible. Foods grown using modern agricultural techniques contain fewer nutrients and minerals.

The twenty-eight countries of the European Union and Russia have banned GMO (genetically modified organisms) foods. Pesticides are genetically engineered into every cell of corn and soy as well as other foods, and there is no information about this on labels in the U.S. Birds and bees are killed by eating GMO corn, which is considered an outrage in Europe. Buying organically grown foods is our only hope of avoiding GMOs, unless you buy organic seeds and grow your own garden.

▲ ▼ ▲

Equipment for the Raw Food Lifestyle Kitchen

First, I must say that the raw and living foods lifestyle can be so easy when eating most foods just as they are found in their natural state, without complicated mixtures. When fresh figs are in season, I love making a meal of them to savor their delicious and unique flavor. However, when transitioning to raw foods or adding a greater percentage of them, nearly everyone wants to create recipes. There are kitchen tools that make this a fun activity, and some of them also help to facilitate digestion.

Blender

This is the main kitchen appliance I use. I own a Vitamix blender, and it is worth every penny I paid for it. I use it to grind seeds and make green smoothies, fresh salad dressings, dips and sauces, raw soups, blended salads, puddings and desserts. I highly recommend purchasing a high-powered blender, a most important piece of equipment for the raw food lifestyle.

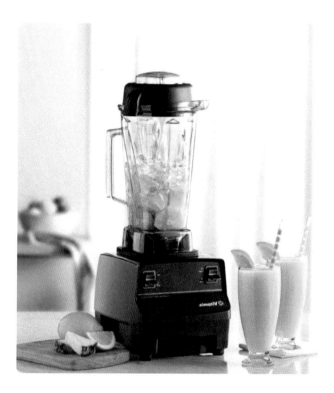

Spiral Slicer, Saladacco, or Spirooli

I love bringing the Spiral Slicer with me when I do speaking engagements. So many people get inspired when I take it out and show how it's used to make delicious veggie pasta of zucchini. The Spiral Slicer makes linguini or ribbon-type pasta noodles. The Spirooli makes a thicker pasta noodle. To purchase a Spiral Slicer, call 201-934-6778 or contact me at karen@superhealthychildren.com.

Food Processor

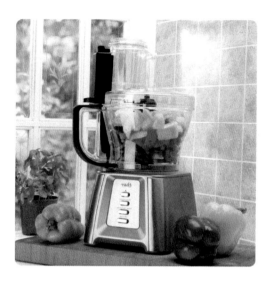

I love making taco fillings, tabouleh, cauliflower "mashed potatoes," banana ice cream and many other raw food dishes in the Villaware food processor. It's best to get a large, 14-cup processor. I purchased the Villaware food processor at Bed, Bath & Beyond for $129 and used a 20%-off coupon that I receive every quarter in the mail. My food processor cost me only a little over $100, and it's definitely the best one I've ever owned.

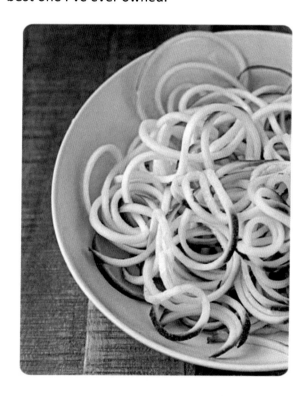

Citrus Juicer

My citrus juicer is the second most used machine when my son is home from college. He loves fresh orange juice and fresh orange-grapefruit-lemon juice blended with pineapple. Sometimes it's difficult to find a good citrus juicer. DiscountJuicers.com/citrus.html is the best website for purchasing kitchen equipment at reasonable prices.

Juice Machine

I bought an auger juicer, the Omega 8004, from John Kohler at http://Discountjuicers.com. This machine is also easy to assemble, allows me to get plenty of juice from leafy green vegetables, is quick to clean up and is reasonably priced.

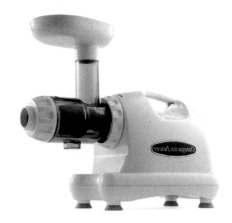

Kitchen Design Tools

Fun kitchen design tools to decorate your fruits and vegetables are pleasant to use, and kids

especially enjoy them. Good knives for cutting fruits and vegetables are also essential tools for the raw food kitchen.

Companies like The Living Light Culinary Arts Institute have an array of handy kitchen supplies available at RawFoodChef.com.
Also check out DiscountJuicers.com

Dehydrator

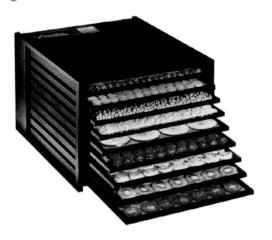

The dehydrator is nice for holidays and special occasions. It heats food at significantly lower temperatures to preserve nutrients but removes the important intrinsic water of fruits and vegetables.

Beautiful Plates, Bowls, Cups and Utensils

These can further capture the nature of raw fruits and vegetables.

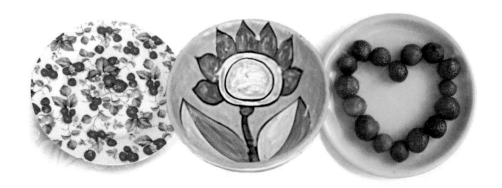

Raw Vegan Recipes for Families

A recent study shows that the risk of stroke increases by 83% when drinking even one soda a day, especially for women. The combo of refined fructose and carbolic acid is lethal. Diet sodas are even worse. Some adolescents are getting 40% of their calories from refined sugars. They can't handle it, and the results are disastrous. Eighty percent of foods sold in America have added refined sugars. Are we doing enough to spread this news? There are beverages in the following recipes that are delicious and health-promoting instead of health-destroying like sodas. I hope you will enjoy these simple healthful recipes for life.

The following Juices, Smoothies, Soups, Sauces, Dips, Cereals, Appetizers, Main Meals, and Party Foods are my gifts for simple healthy eating for your family. The recipes are my creation unless noted that it's shared by another raw vegan expert or chef.

Juices

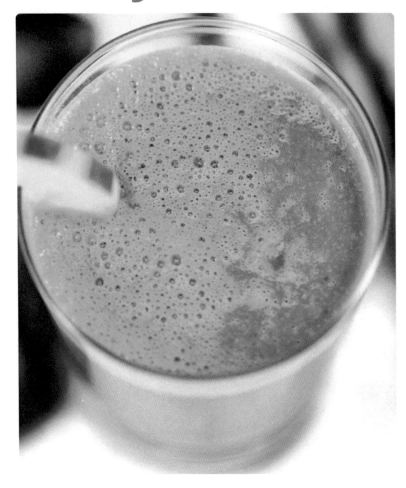

The Healing Asthma Green Juice

1 to 3 carrots
1 or 2 cucumbers,
    sliced down the middle lengthwise
1 large bunch celery
4 to 6 leaves of kale

Juice the carrot, cucumber and celery, then juice the kale.

As a variation, some days I use one Granny Smith apple instead of a carrot, or one small lemon and a small piece of ginger. Sometimes I like to add delicious pea shoots I get from the local organic farmer.

Nutrients in greens, such as kale and spinach, are more easily absorbed when using the auger juicers.

Pineapple Greens

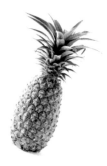

¼ large pineapple
4 Romaine lettuce leaves
¼ cup parsley

Cut the skin off the pineapple and then chop into chunks that will fit into a juicer. Juice all ingredients and pour into elegant glasses.

Popeye's Juice

1 cup spinach
¼ cup arugula
6 carrots
¼ cup cilantro or parsley

Slice carrots into pieces that fit into the juice machine. Juice all ingredients and serve in beautiful glasses.

Heavenly Cocktail

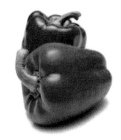

2 stalks celery
1 cucumber
1 tomato
1 red bell pepper

Juice and enjoy!

Juicing greens provides alkalinity to the body and supplies easy to assimilate vitamins and minerals.

Orange, Cucumber and Celery Juice

Shared by Carissa Leventis-Cox of
MamaInTheKitchen.com

4 cups freshly squeezed orange juice
3 cucumbers
4 celery stalks

In the autumn, use sour oranges. In the winter, use Washington Navels. In the spring, use sweet oranges, tangelos or temple oranges.

Juice the cucumbers and celery. You should have about 4 cups in total. Combine 4 cups of orange juice with 4 cups of the green juice.

Voilà! A delightful drink! Use less orange juice for "Superhero Green Juice Guzzlers" and more when the kids aren't into Superheroes! This is easily my son's favorite drink these days. It is best in summer or autumn, when cucumbers are in season.

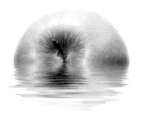

Pink Juice

Shared by Margrieta Lasmane

5 apples, chopped
2 medium beets, chopped

Juice for beautiful pink juice.

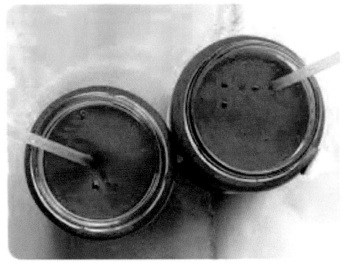

Jasmine's Citrus Juice

Shared by Margrieta Lasmane

Tangerine
Oranges
Grapefruit
Lime

Juice all ingredients with citrus juicer.
This is a beautiful and delicious juice!

{ *Rinse your mouth with water after drinking the juice.* }

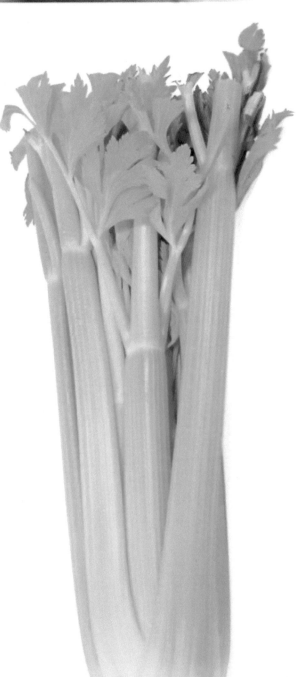

My Favorite Morning Juice

Shared by Margrieta Lasmane

Granny Smith apple
Cucumber
Celery

Juice all ingredients.

Green Smoothies

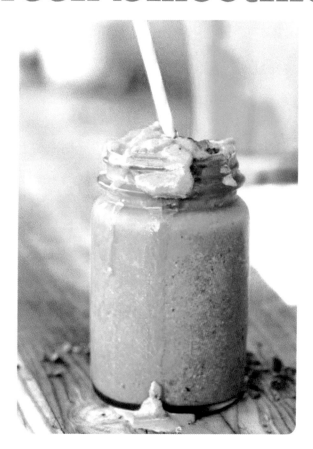

Read *5 Tips for Getting Your Kids to Eat Their Leafy Greens* (see page 76) and more in the *Additional Readings* section.

Wild Edible Dream

1 apple
2 big chunks of pineapple
1 cup lambsquarters (wild spinach)
2 cups water

Blend until smooth. *Yum!*

Splendid Smoothie

2 cups watermelon
1 mango
7 Romaine lettuce leaves

Blend together until smooth.

Yummy Collard Summer Smoothie

1 cup raspberries
1 frozen banana
4 to 5 collard leaves
3 nectarines
2 cups water

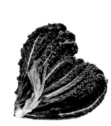

Blend all ingredients until smooth.

Dandelion Applesauce

1 small to medium bunch dandelion leaves
3 Granny Smith apples

Blend together until smooth.

This green applesauce feels so nourishing!

Emerald Smoothie

1 banana, chopped
1 mango peeled, pitted and chopped
6 lacinato kale leaves
2 cups of water

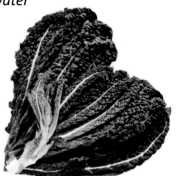

Blend banana and mango and then kale and water. Blend again until smooth.

Blueberry Smoothie

1 banana
1 ½ cups fresh or frozen blueberries
2 large handfuls of lambsquarter
    (wild spinach) or spinach

Blend together until smooth.

Green 'n' Clean Smoothie

Shared by Brian Rossiter of *Fruit-Powered.com*

3 ripe bananas
4-5 Romaine lettuce leaves

Blend all ingredients for creamy, thick smoothie consistency.

Variation: Change your greens—use green or red leaf lettuce, for example, for smooth and delicate green smoothies, and enjoy your delicious meal!

Family Green Smoothie

Shared by the Evans-Mear family

1 ¼ cups water
1 ripe banana
2 celery ribs without the leaves
4 dandelion leaves (alternatively use spinach,
    sunflower greens or kale)
6 lettuce leaves
1 heaping teaspoon chia seeds

{ *We grind them at home just before using for
freshness, lower cost and to avoid rancidity.* }

Blend all ingredients and enjoy!

Variation: In the winter, we add frozen blueberries or strawberries that are frozen in the summer after purchasing them locally grown— about ½ cup.

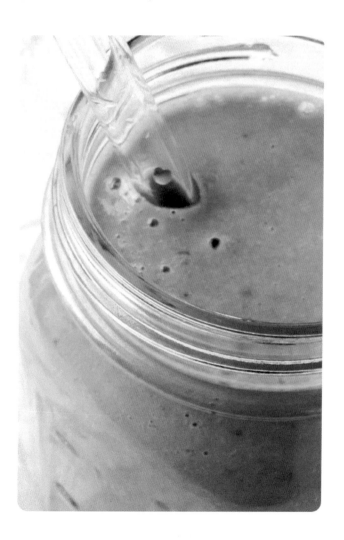

Piña Colada Green Smoothie

2 bananas, chopped
Big chunk of pineapple, chopped
2 large handfuls of baby spinach
    or Romaine lettuce
2 cups of water or 2 cups of watermelon

Blend all ingredients until smooth.

Our Pirate's Smoothie

*Shared by Carissa Leventis-Cox of
MamaInTheKitchen.com*

2 young coconuts
1 ripe pineapple, peeled and cut into chunks

Place pineapple chunks, coconut water and meat of the two coconuts in a high-speed blender and puree. This is heavenly, especially after a day at the beach!

Creamy Strawberry-Plantain Green Smoothie

*Shared by Carissa Leventis-Cox of
MamaInTheKitchen.com*

2 really ripe, soft and black plantains, peeled
1 cup freshly squeezed orange juice
1 cup water
1 pint strawberries or fruits in season
6 or more cups of greens

Blend all ingredients in a high-speed blender.

Plantains create lovely creamy drinks. For those days when you are really hungry, these smoothies are creamier than those made with regular bananas. Plantains are an excellent source of potassium, magnesium and vitamins B6 and C.

Very Cherry Smoothie

Shared by Carissa Leventis-Cox of
MamaInTheKitchen.com

2 pitted dates
3 bananas
2 cups freshly squeezed orange juice
16 ounces pitted cherries
6 cups kale, stemmed

{ *I sometimes freeze my bananas*
for a cooler drink in the summer. }

Puree in a high-speed blender.

Cherries seem to be the "in" fruit these days. They are a wonderful fruit for cleansing the blood, detoxifying acids in the body and strengthening our hearts and plasma. One cup of cherries contains 16% of our daily need for Vitamin C and also contains beta-carotene, potassium, magnesium and melatonin.

Cantaloupe Sorbet Smoothie

Shared by Kristina Carrillo-Bucaram of
RawFullyOrganic.com and FullyRaw.com

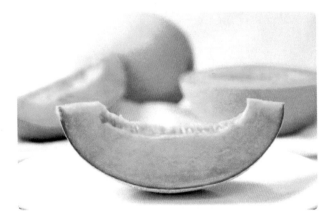

This recipe celebrates our first cantaloupes of the summer season! Melons are best eaten alone for digestion, and this recipe is easy and true to proper food combining! Best when savored in the sun! Enjoy this cool treat!

Unlimited cantaloupe (if you eat enough,
    this can be eaten as a full meal)
Few sprigs of mint
Blueberries (optional)

{ *Wait until your cantaloupe ripens properly.*
If you wait until it is soft at the end and smells potent, the taste will be significantly sweeter! }

1   Cut the skin off the cantaloupe. Get as close to the edge as you can as to avoid waste. Cut the cantaloupe into chunks.

2   Freeze the cantaloupe in a glass container. When frozen, place the chunks into a food processor with a few sprigs of mint.

3   Scoop out the sorbet and top with a few more mint sprigs and a blueberry.

Orange You Glad You Tried This Smoothie a.k.a. Vitamin C Smoothie

Shared by Lisa Montgomery of
LivingDynamically.com

2 to 3 oranges, peeled
3 bananas, peeled
1 young Thai coconut, milk and water

Open the young Thai coconut carefully. *

{ *If you are not sure how to do this, watch this:*
YouTube.com/watch?v=3caGfCpIAUw
and learn how to safely open a Thai coconut! }

Combine ingredients in a high-speed blender until well combined. For a thicker smoothie leave as is. For a thinner consistency add a little water.

Coconut water is extremely hydrophilic and contains the best electrolytes on the planet.

LJ's Creamy Banana Shake

Shared by Linda Joy Rose, Ph.D., of
RawFusionLiving.com

This is a wonderful non-dairy shake when you are craving something rich and creamy. Very appealing to kids. Also makes a great meal replacement.

4 cups water
3 ripe bananas (fresh or frozen)
1 cup sprouted and dried buckwheat*
2 Tablespoons chia seeds
1 Tablespoon lucuma
1 teaspoon cinnamon
1 ½ teaspoon alcohol-free vanilla extract
    or 1 vanilla bean

Soak buckwheat for 6-8 hours and sprout for a day. Dry in dehydrator at 105 degrees. Grind buckwheat and chia seeds to a fine meal in coffee grinder.

Optional: Add 1-2 tablespoons of raw green powder.

Add everything to your blender container and blend until rich and creamy.

Green Fairy's Lemonade

Shared by Linda Joy Rose, Ph.D., of
RawFusionLiving.com

½ head of leafy greens
5 stalks kale (use only the leaves)
1 lemon
1 apple
½-1 inch fresh ginger
½ cucumber
½ cup fresh or frozen pineapple
Filtered water

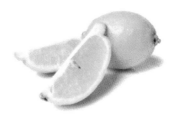

Place greens in blender first, then add other ingredients, blend and enjoy.

I drank this mixture every day for the first 6 weeks when I went raw. If you don't like the foaminess of the kale, you can also run this through your juicer. Save the pulp because it's very tasty.

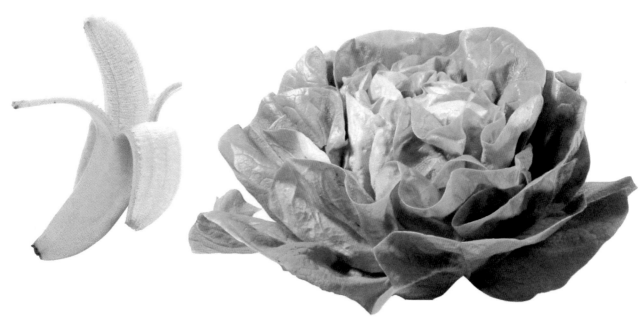

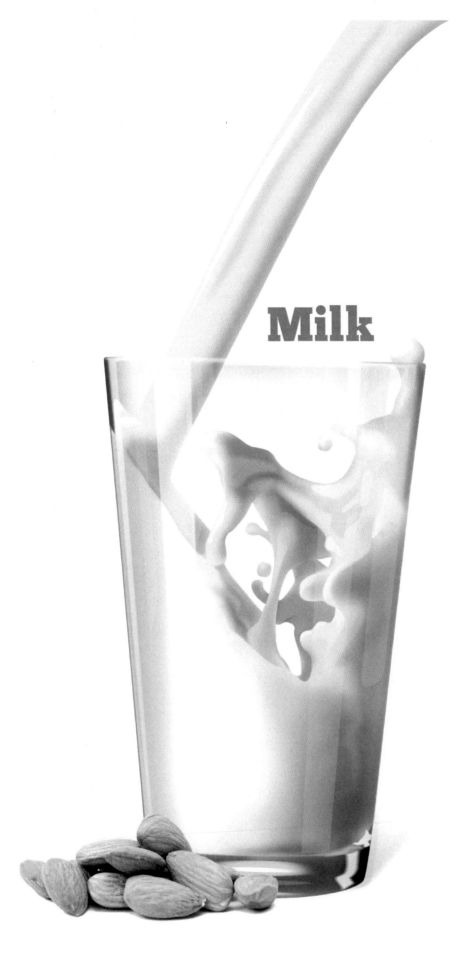

Milk

Pumpkin Seed Milk

Shared by Priscilla Soligo of RawthenticFood.com

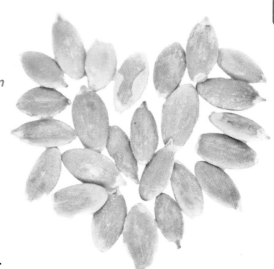

½ cup pumpkin seeds (presoaked 4 hours,
    rinsed and drained)
2 cups filtered water
3 large pitted Medjool dates
1 teaspoon alcohol-free vanilla extract
    or 12 drops vanilla by Medicine Flower

Blend all ingredients in a high-speed blender.
Strain milk through a nut milk bag into a separate bowl.

Almond Milk

1 cup raw almonds, soaked overnight and then rinsed
4 cups water
3-4 dates, soaked for 20 minutes
    or, for less problematic food combining, use 5 tamarind seeds in place of each date

Blend soaked almonds and water until smooth. Strain the milk through a sprout bag or cheesecloth into a container, squeezing the bag to get the most milk. Pour the strained milk back into the blender, add the dates or tamarind seeds and blend again until smooth.

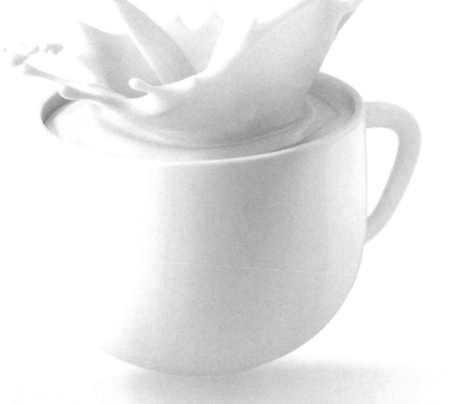

Cereals

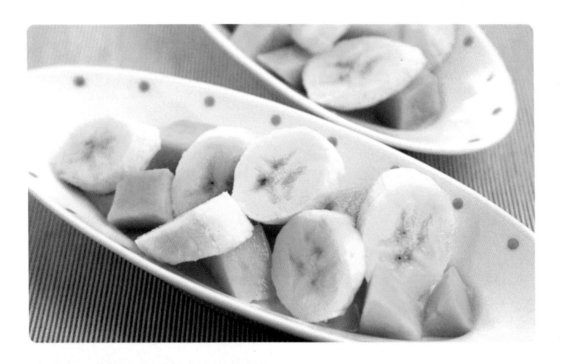

The following yummy and warming cereal recipes, especially nice during those cold winter months in northern climates, provide comfort without the toxicity of processed, packaged cereals cooked at high enough temperatures that cause acrylamide to form. To learn more on this topic, see my book *Creating Healthy Children,* available at SuperHealthyChildren.com.

BAT Cereal:
Banana, Apple and Tahini

This was the delicious cereal replacement that originally got my kids and me off of the processed, packaged cereals. It was very satisfying on cold winter mornings, and in the summer we would replace the apple with a peach or a nectarine. Tahini (sesame seed paste) with bananas is not an ideal combination, but it's miles better than the totally indigestible typical, processed cereals and bagels that are standard fare in the morning.

2 bananas
1 apple
1 teaspoon of tahini

Mash bananas, mix in a scoop of raw tahini, and top with small, coarsely chopped apple pieces and mix to combine.

My family has loved this yummy cereal replacement for many years.

Mango Heaven

1 large mango, peeled and sliced
2 bananas
1 frozen banana
1 lime

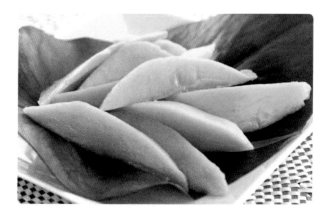

Put the mango and banana through a juicer that has a blank plate. Alternately, place the mango and bananas in a high-powered blender and add a little water just to get the mixture moving. Pour into a pretty bowl and squeeze lime juice on the mixture. Serve on top of fresh greens.

Chia Seed Pudding

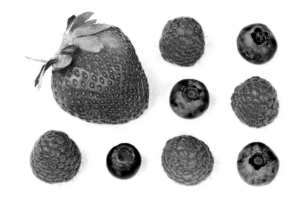

4 Tablespoons chia seeds
1 cup almond milk (see page 29)
1 cup fresh juicy fruit

Chop fresh fruit into a bowl. Add milk and chia seeds and let it sit for 10 minutes. Blueberries and/or raspberries make a nice addition.

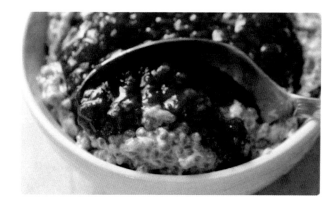

TIP: In cold weather, instead of nut milk, add warm water to the chia seeds to make a nice winter breakfast that is quick to prepare.

Windsor's Yummy Fruit and Raisin Cereal

Shared by 16-year-old Windsor Griffing of RawFoodCentral.com

For almond-blueberry milk:*
10-15 almonds, soaked
2 ripe bananas
1 cup fresh or thawed frozen blueberries
2 cups distilled water

1   Place almonds in a high-speed blender with water, 1 banana and 1 cup blueberries. Blend on high for 30-60 seconds.

For cereal:
1 apple
1 pear
1 cup fresh or thawed frozen blueberries
1 cup raisins or more if you like

{ *Soaking raisins first is always better but not a must.* }

2   Chop and place all ingredients in a large serving bowl and toss.

3   Pour the *almond-blueberry milk* over your fruit and enjoy!

TIP: *If you like a crunchy cereal, dice 2 stalks of celery into small pieces and add in with fruit.*

*See also other raw vegan milk recipes on page 28.

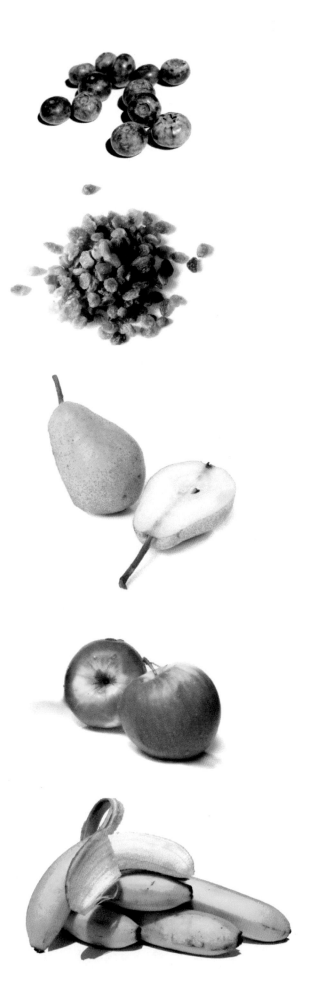

Dressings, Sauces, Salsas and Marinades

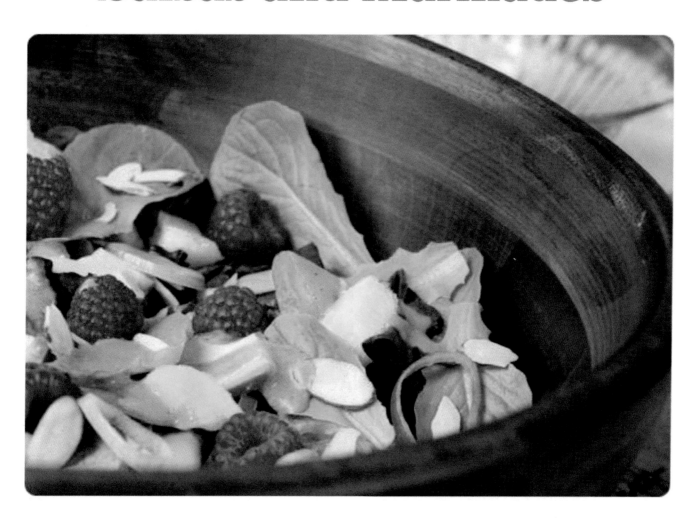

Luscious Thousand Island Dressing

⅓ cup pine nuts, soaked 2 hours
¼ cup fresh lemon juice
2 Roma tomatoes, chopped
¼ cup fresh basil, chopped
½ cup parsley, chopped
2 stalks celery, chopped

Blend until smooth. Serve as a dressing or dip.

If your kids just need a sweet, low fat dressing on their salads, try **Mango Raspberry Dressing.**

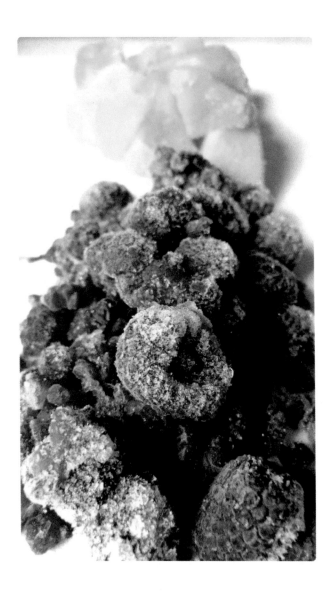

Mango Raspberry Dressing

6 organic mangos
    (peeled, with the pits discarded)
6 ounces raspberries

Blend until smooth, and pour over a large lettuce or spinach salad.

Fresh Cilantro Dressing

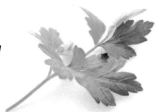

½ cup celery juice
½ cup fresh cilantro, chopped
¼ cup lemon juice
2 Tablespoons raw tahini

Blend all ingredients until smooth.

Creamy Cucumber-Dill Dressing

See My Favorite High Green Salad with Creamy Cucumber-Dill Dressing *page 53*

2 to 3 ounces macadamia nuts
1 ½ cups cucumbers, peeled and chopped
2 stalks celery, chopped
2 soft or soaked pitted dates
Juice of ½ lemon
½ cup fresh dill

Blend all ingredients until smooth and creamy.

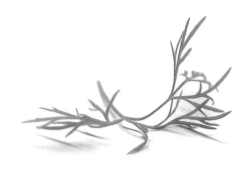

Creamy Avocado Dressing

1 small avocado
1 red bell pepper
2 scallions (green onions), chopped
4 Tablespoons lemon juice
½ cup water
1 teaspoon ground cumin

Blend all ingredients until smooth and creamy.

Blueberry and Macadamia Dressing

Shared by Dr. Timothy Trader

Most kids generally have problems eating salads because they are used to the typical diet. This simple, sweet dressing recipe most kids love instead of the common "savory" dressings of the usual raw recipes. It combines well with lettuce and tomatoes.

10 ounces organic blueberries
(fresh, or frozen and thawed)
¼ ounce organic chia seeds
1 ½ ounces of shelled organic macadamia nuts
¼ cup water

Blend blueberries and water until smooth, then add the chia seeds and macadamia nuts until smooth again. Pour over a large dinner salad of lettuce and tomatoes.

I have included fats with this dressing because I believe kids, especially younger ones, need some fat.

The chia seeds increase the Omega-3 essential fatty acids and help thicken the dressing.

The nuts also give the creamy sensation we all crave; yet, in these recipes, fat is not found in excessive amounts as it is in so many raw recipes.

Zippy Red Pepper-Ginger Dressing

Shared by Nomi Shannon RawGourmet.com

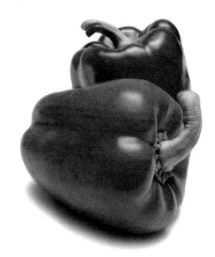

2 red bell peppers, juiced or diced
¼ cup chopped parsley
1-inch piece ginger root, grated
2 teaspoons lemon juice
1-2 teaspoons ground flaxseeds (optional)*
Water (optional)

*To grind flaxseeds, place them in a clean electric coffee grinder and process them until powdered.

TIP 1: Red bell pepper juice gives this dressing a lovely red color and a light, sweet flavor. If you are pressed for time, toss the peppers into the blender without juicing them. Dice peppers, and put them into the blender, a few pieces at a time, until the blades "catch" and liquefy them. This will result in a thicker dressing that contains bits of pepper skin, but it will cut your preparation time in half.

In a blender, combine the red bell pepper juice, parsley, ginger and lemon juice. Blend well. To thin the dressing, add water. To thicken it, add ground flaxseeds. Yields approximately ¾-1 cup.

TIP 2: Alter this recipe with half a cup of carrot juice in place of the pepper juice.

Apple Sauce

Young children especially love this.

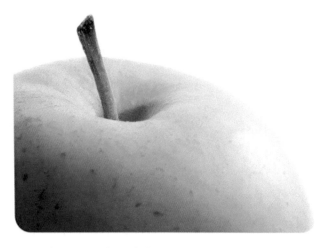

2 apples, cored and diced
3 dates, pitted
Dash of cinnamon
Water to blend

Blend all ingredients until smooth and serve immediately!

Lemon-Date Sauce

See Kale-Beet-Apple Combo Delish page 55

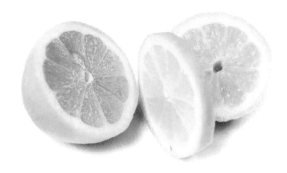

A friend told me she had been to a potluck where this elegant combination was served. I tried it during a Raw Food Challenge class I hosted, and everyone loved it.

Juice of 1 large lemon
3 small soaked dates
    or 2 large soaked Medjool dates

Blend the juice of the lemon with the dates. Add some of the soak water to blend if necessary. Pour *Lemon-Date Sauce* over the *Kale-Beet-Apple Combo Delish* dish and combine.

Tomatillo Sauce

See Romaine Burritos page 56

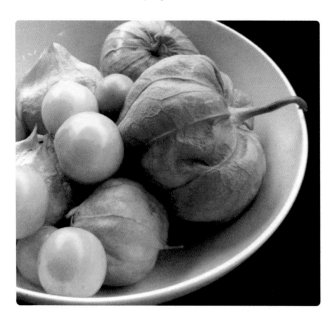

2 cups tomatillos, chopped
⅓ cup cilantro, chopped
3 Tablespoons soaked raisins
¼ avocado
1 clove garlic, minced (optional)
3 Tablespoons lemon juice

Use the "S" blade to process all ingredients in the food processor until it's a chunky salsa.

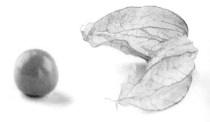

Lemon Tahini Sauce

See Pineapple Coleslaw page 56

2 Tablespoons raw tahini
Juice of one lemon
1 Tablespoon water
½ teaspoon ground cumin

Mix all ingredients in a bowl using a whisk or fork. Pour sauce over the *Pineapple Coleslaw* and mix thoroughly.

Mango Tomato Salsa

2 large mangos, peeled and diced
2 heaping Tablespoons red onion, chopped
2 medium tomatoes, diced
Juice from 1 lime
⅓ cup cilantro, minced

Mix all ingredients in a medium size bowl.

Variation: Add a small piece of jalapeño if a spicier salsa is desired.

Tomato Salsa

See Romaine Burritos page 56

4 tomatoes, diced
⅓ cup cilantro, finely chopped
2 scallions, finely chopped
2 Tablespoons lemon juice
Small pinch cayenne

Mix in a bowl and serve.

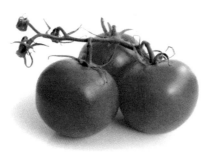

Tomato Marinade for Kabobs

See Kabobs page 62

2 large heirloom tomatoes
1 Tablespoon lemon juice
7 fresh basil leaves
    or 1 Tablespoon fresh oregano
5 black olives, chopped

Blend all marinade ingredients and pour over kabobs. Marinate for 3 hours at room temperature, occasionally moving around to cover with the marinade, or marinate overnight in a refrigerator.

Marinara Sauce for Zucchini Linguini

See Zucchini Linguini page 51

2 large whole ripe tomatoes chopped
8-10 soaked sun-dried tomatoes
2 soaked dates (optional)
10 fresh basil leaves
Handful fresh oregano leaves (optional)

Blend tomatoes, sun-dried tomatoes, dates, fresh basil and oregano until slightly chunky.

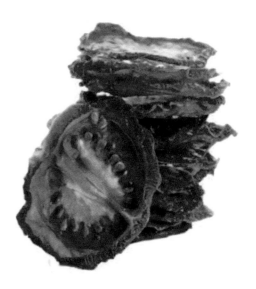

Thai Sauce for Thai Pasta

See Thai Pasta page 51

1 cup freshly squeezed orange juice
⅔ cup soaked almonds (½ cup before soaking)
1 teaspoon curry powder

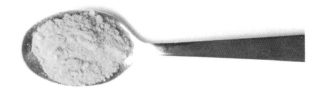

Soak ½ cup almonds overnight, discarding soak water in the morning. Blendall ingredients until smooth and stir into zucchini linguini.

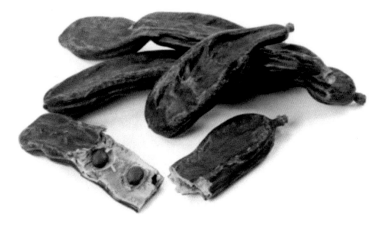

"Chocolate" Heaven

This is delicious over fresh fruit or banana ice cream.

1 cup raw carob powder
½ cup dates, pitted and soaked for 20 minutes
1 teaspoon vanilla powder

Blend this sauce until smooth. Add a little water if too thick.

{ *Brush and floss after eating dried fruits such as dates.* }

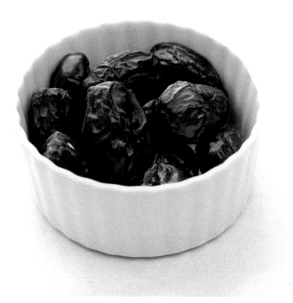

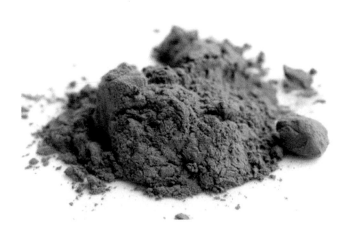

Dips and Pâtés

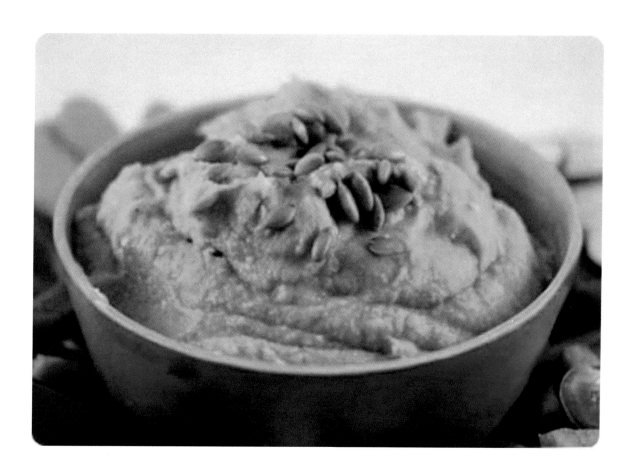

Red Pepper Cheeze Sauce or Dip

This sauce or dip can also be a dressing for a large salad. Play with the amount of water and lemon juice to make it the consistency of your choice.

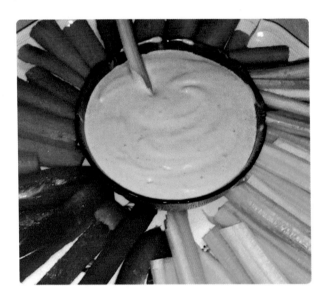

Did you know ...

Did you know that many cheeses are <u>not</u> <u>vegetarian</u> since they contain <u>rennet,</u> which comes from the <u>stomachs</u> of calves taken from dairy cows and slaughtered within a few days of birth? There are vegetarian forms of rennet, but it is most often sourced from veal calves. So, basically, cheese is made by mixing cow milk with pieces of her dead babies' stomachs. This is what we commonly say "Yes" to when we purchase or consume cow milk products. The *Red Pepper Cheeze Sauce or Dip* recipe tastes cheesy but doesn't come from animals. Nuts are not meant to be eaten in huge quantities, but some of the preceding "cheeze" sauce over a salad or over zucchini pasta or as a dip will provide a nice transition from cow cheese.

—An article from a local newspaper, Dec 29, '10
"Cow milk formula leads to obesity."

1 cup macadamia nuts,
 soaked 3 hours and rinsed
2 Tablespoons lemon juice
1 red bell pepper, chopped
½ teaspoon dulse flakes*
½ cup water or more for desired consistency

{ **Dulse is a seaweed that adds a nice salty taste to this recipe.* }

Blend macadamia nuts by themselves until finely ground. Add remaining ingredients and blend until smooth.

Macadamia nuts have a high fat content, and therefore this recipe is meant for several people or a party. It could also be served over Zucchini Linguini (see page 51).

TIP: *For heat and Mexican flavor, add a small amount of chili powder.*

No Bean Hummus

2 cups peeled zucchini, chopped
½ cup hulled sesame seeds
Juice of one lemon
1 clove garlic (optional)
1 teaspoon paprika

Blend all ingredients until smooth.

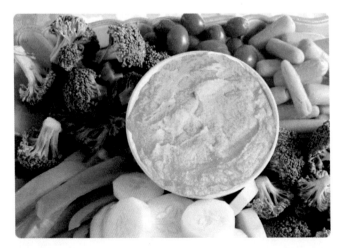

Pumpkin Seed Pâté

Pumpkin seeds are an excellent source of zinc, protein, magnesium, manganese and other nutrients, and wonderful for growing children. Sesame seeds are an excellent source of calcium, copper, manganese, iron and other nutrients.

¾ cup pumpkin seeds,
     soaked overnight and rinsed
¾ cup white sesame seeds, soaked and rinsed
2 Tablespoons fresh basil, minced
2 Tablespoons fresh parsley, minced
Juice of 1 lime

Begin to process the seeds in a food processor with the "S" blade. Then add basil, parsley and lime and continue to process. Garnish with basil leaves, parsley sprigs, quartered cherry tomatoes and/or diced red bell pepper.

Eat with red bell peppers.* Take 1 or 2 scoops and serve atop a large green salad. Will last in a refrigerator for 3 days.

*Eat red bell peppers instead of the green ones. Green peppers have not yet ripened and have 3 times less Vitamin C as well as beta-carotene.

Root Veggies Pâté

This is one of my favorite dishes to place over a large green salad for a complete meal.

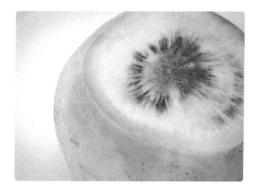

3 medium carrots, chopped
1 stalk celery, chopped
1 medium rutabaga, peeled and chopped
Juice of one lemon
2 Tablespoons raw tahini (sesame seed paste)
2 Tablespoons fresh dill or thyme, chopped

Process carrots, celery and rutabaga in food processor until finely ground. Add lemon juice, tahini, and dill. Process until it reaches the consistency of a smooth pâté.

Carrot-Ginger Dip

Try with Nori Rolls, see page 57

½ cup fresh carrot juice
2 Tablespoons fresh lemon juice
4 Tablespoons purified water
2 teaspoons fresh ginger, grated

Blend all ingredients and refrigerate until served.

Rosemary Cream Cheeze

Shared by Anna Chmielewska of SweetVeganNature.com

1 cup buckwheat, soaked overnight
1 avocado
½ cup zucchini, quartered
1 celery stalk, quartered
1 shallot, halved
2 Tablespoons fresh rosemary,
     minced or very well-chopped
1 Medjool date
Juice from 2 lemons

Mix all ingredients in a food processor until smooth. Add more avocado for creamier and more lemon juice for runnier consistency. Eat with lettuce leaves and chopped veggies!

Simple Appetizers
and Raw Finger Foods

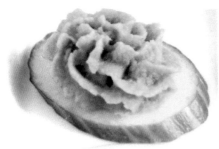 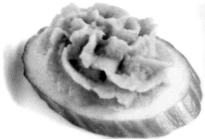 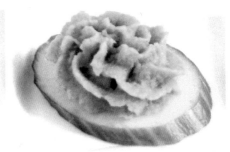

Pine Nut Lasagna Appetizers

This works well as an appetizer and is nice to set out for the holidays. It's especially delicious when heirloom tomatoes are available. My children, Gabriela and Marco, were preparing this dish when they were videotaped for a show called "Highlighting Vegetarian Children" for Nickelodeon Kids News in 2000.

½ cup pine nuts or macadamia nuts
2 tomatoes

Using the "S" blade in a mini food processor, grind ½ cup of nuts until they look like Parmesan cheese. Thinly slice two large, beautiful ripe tomatoes and prepare by placing one tomato slice on a plate, then a thin layer of nut cheese, then another tomato slice and then nut cheese again. Make as many layers as you like.

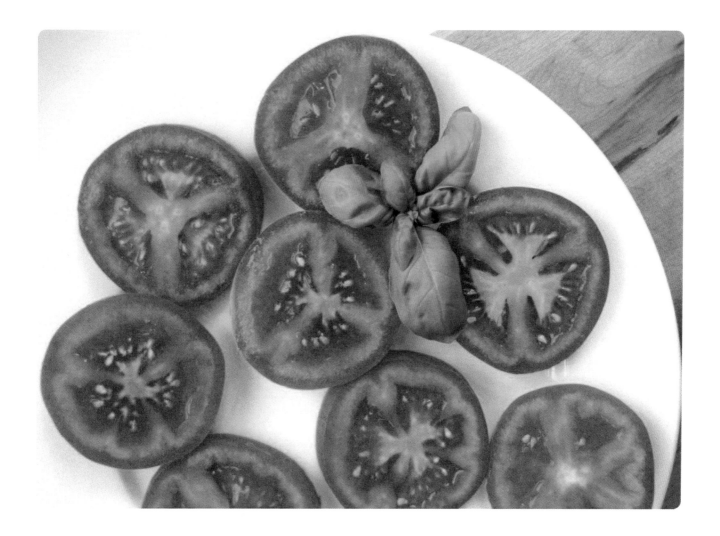

Stuffed Herb Pesto Holiday Appetizers

Dehydration time: 3 to 4 hours

These are delicious also when not dehydrated. Pesto can be made in advance and marinated overnight in a refrigerator.

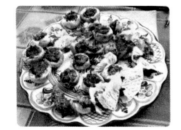

⅓ cup pine nuts, soaked 20 minutes
½ cup parsley, chopped
½ cup basil, chopped
½ cup cilantro, chopped
1 tomato, chopped
Zucchini rounds
Bell pepper pieces
Mushroom caps
2 small cloves fresh garlic (optional), minced

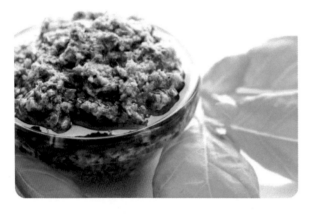

First, grind the pine nuts in a food processor. Add the garlic and fresh herbs and process until finely chopped. Spread pesto on each mushroom, pepper or zucchini piece and dehydrate at 105 degrees for 3 to 4 hours. For a final touch, a slice of olive can be added to the top of each dehydrated pesto appetizer before serving.

Cucumber Sandwiches

One Roma tomato, cut into thin slices
One cucumber, sliced thinly

Fresh basil, coarsely chopped
Raw walnut butter or raw tahini
   or any nut or seed butter

Spread walnut butter or tahini on thin cucumber slices. Place a slice of tomato, topped with the chopped basil, and then cover with another slice of cucumber to make a sandwich. Continue with the remainder of slices.

Stuffed Tomato or Stuffed Pepper

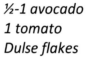

½-1 avocado
1 tomato
Dulse flakes
Juice of half a lemon or one lime

Mash ½-1 avocado in a bowl. Cut off the top of the tomato and cut along the inner edges to scoop out the pulp. Add the tomato pulp to the mashed avocado, add lemon juice to taste and fill the empty tomato with the mixture. Replace the tomato top.

Variation: Scoop the filling into a red bell pepper that has been carved out and deseeded. My daughter, Gabriela, grew up relishing this simple recipe.

Cucumber or Zucchini Snacks

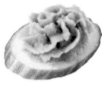

1 cucumber, sliced
Dip, Cheeze or Pâté of choice, see pages 40-41

Prepare the topping of choice and, using piping bag or just a fork, create nice spiral decorations on top of each cucumber slice.

Cucumber "Dogs"

1 cucumber
1 mango, diced
1 tomato, diced

These are especially nice during the warmer weather when you can get local cucumbers and heirloom tomatoes.

Slice the cucumber in half lengthwise and scoop out seeds to make a hollow area in each half of the cucumber. Fill the indentation with the mango and tomato mixture.

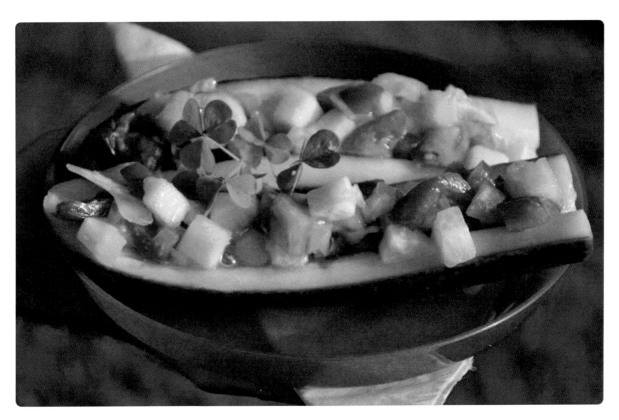

Ants on a Log

Celery stalks
Raw unsalted almond butter, walnut butter, pecan butter, or pistachio butter (I do not recommend the use of peanut butter.)*
Raisins

Spread a thin layer of raw nut butter on celery stalks and dot with raisins.

Did you know ...

*Peanuts are legumes, not nuts. Peanut butter is almost always roasted and contains aflatoxins—one of the most potent toxic molds that occurs naturally.

Simple Raw Soups

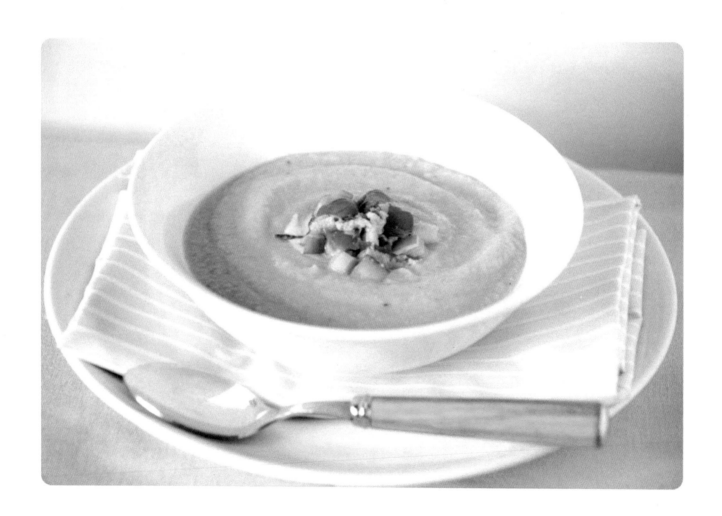

Spring Garden Soup

2 large tomatoes, chopped
1 carrot, chopped
½ sweet red pepper
   (green pepper is unripe)
½ zucchini
½ avocado
1 small shallot
Juice of 1 lime

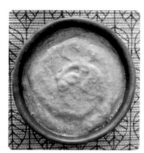

Blend until smooth.

I make this soup at my "Raw Food Fun for Families" class, and it's always a big hit.

Gazpacho Soup

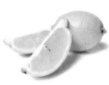

5 medium tomatoes, chopped finely
1 red pepper, deseeded and chopped finely
1 cucumber, finely chopped
1 small avocado, peeled and chopped
¼ cup fresh cilantro, chopped
½ cup fresh basil, chopped
½ cup ripe pineapple (optional)
¾ cup water
¼ cup lemon or lime juice

Combine all ingredients in a large bowl and mix. Pour half into a food processor and pulse. Return processed mix to the bowl and mix with remaining ingredients.

Tomato Vegetable Soup

Shared by Dr. Timothy Trader

3 large organic tomatoes, quartered
1 cup diced organic celery
1 medium organic cucumber, chopped
½ cup diced organic red bell peppers

1 cup sweet tamarind,* shell removed
   and deseeded
½ cup chopped organic tomatillos
½ cup shredded organic Chinese cabbage

*Fresh organic tamarind is almost impossible to find, though most farmers do not find the need for chemicals.

Blend the tomatoes, cucumber and ½ cup of the celery. After your blend is smooth, add and blend in the tamarind. Pour over rest of ingredients and serve.

Note that because I follow the precepts of correct food combining, I don't include starchy carrots or corn.

Creamy Butter-Me-Up Soup

Shared by Priscilla Soligo of RawthenticFood.com

Such a bright and beautiful comfort food soup!

2 cups butternut squash, chopped
¼ cup young Thai coconut pulp*
1 cup young Thai coconut water
2 Tablespoon hemp seeds
1 teaspoon curry powder (mild-no heat)
1 Tablespoon onion powder (optional)
½ cup filtered water,
      or, as needed for desired consistency

*Open a young Thai coconut and put water aside. Remove the white pulp inside. 1 coconut usually yields approximately ¼ cup pulp.

In a high-speed blender, blend all ingredients together until well-incorporated and smooth. Add in more water until desired consistency has been achieved. Serve immediately.

This soup will keep for up to 2 days in an airtight container in a refrigerator.

Creamy Carrot-Beet Soup

Shared by Brandi Rollins of
RawFoodsOnABudget.com

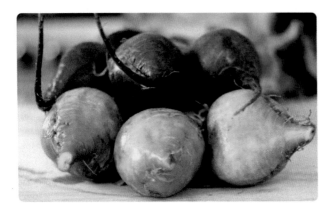

1 medium apple
¼ cup water
½ medium beet
1 medium sized organic carrot
1 teaspoon lemon juice
2 dates
6 walnuts, Brazil nuts, or pecans

Peel and cube the apple, beet and carrot. Using a high-speed blender or food processor, blend the apple cubes and water until liquefied. Add the remaining ingredients and blend until the soup is creamy (about 1-3 minutes in a food processor).

Tip 1: If you are using a food processor, after processing, spoon the slightly chunky soup into a masticating juicer with a blank screen (the one with no holes). The juicer will then chew up the small chunks. Enjoy!

Tip 2: You can easily warm this soup for the winter months by blending until slightly warmed or warm it on the stove. Just keep your finger in the soup to prevent it from getting too warm.

Sweet n Sassy Tomato Soup!

Shared by Curtis Griffing of RawFoodCentral.com

2 cups freshly squeezed orange juice,
    from organic oranges
8 large, delicious ripe tomatoes
1 pound organic Swiss chard

Cut off the top ⅓ of the tomatoes and blend them with the orange juice and all the Swiss chard, using a tamper or celery stalk to press the Swiss chard into the blender.

Dice the remaining tomatoes into small cubes, and mix into the sweet and salty chard goodness.

Serious yum!

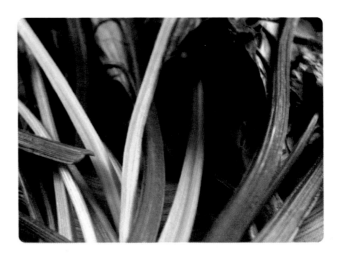

Green Soup with Blueberries

Shared by Margrieta Lasmane

2 mangos
1 apple
1 orange
2 handfuls spinach (variation could be kale
    or celery without the leaves)
Freshly squeezed orange juice
Handful blueberries

Blend all ingredients and pour into a bowl. Add the blueberries on top and serve.

Sweet Celery Soup
with Blueberry Crunchies

Shared by Margrieta Lasmane

6 stalks celery
3 bananas
1 mango
4 apples
½ cup water
Fresh blueberries

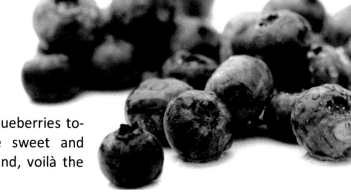

Blend all the ingredients except blueberries together. Then add some of the sweet and crunchy blueberries to the soup and, voilà the yummy dish is ready. Enjoy!

Cucumber Soup

Shared by Julia Lucas (Raw Julia) of RawJulia.com

2 cucumbers
1 avocado
Juice of 2 lemons or to taste
1 clove of garlic (optional)
1 ½ cups of water
1 teaspoon of curry powder
½ cup fresh basil leaves

Place all ingredients in a blender. You may add or substitute fresh oregano, sage, mint, parsley, chives or scallions. This soup is great chilled.

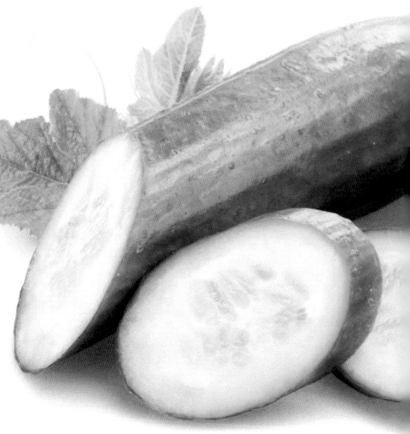

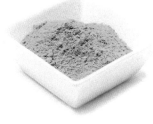

Main Dishes
and Salads

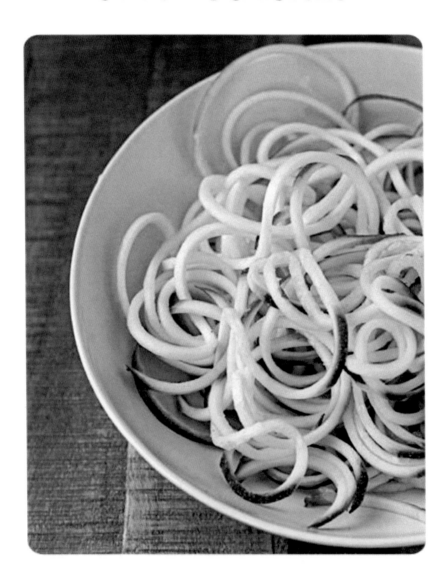

Growing Up on Pasta

*A*s a child growing up, I used to love spaghetti covered with a thick canned tomato sauce and sprinkle it generously with Parmesan cheese. Pasta and bread were the most difficult processed food addictions for me to give up when I turned to the raw food lifestyle for my sustenance. The night before going 100% raw, I consumed an entire loaf of almond-butter-and-jelly sandwiches on whole wheat bread!

The processed and cooked starches in pastas and breads can only provide empty calories since their enzymes and vitamins have been destroyed by heat and their minerals have been removed in the refining process. Pastas and breads are acid-forming, devoid of electrical charge or life force and require cooking and processing in order to be eaten. Consuming large amounts of cooked starches can cause candida, chronic fatigue, diabetes and various other physical problems. Pastas, breads and chips are so demineralized that regular consumption of these processed foods does not permit enough minerals such as calcium to be absorbed.

Instead of the spaghetti I grew up on, living on raw foods since 1994, I eat zucchini pasta instead. The zucchini pasta is made by placing chunks of zucchini in a small, child-friendly, non-electrical kitchen device called the Spiral Slicer (formerly known as Saladacco) and cranking out zucchini linguini. A variety of sauces can be added to give it the familiar pasta and tomato sauce, pasta and Alfredo sauce, or pasta pesto. Below are a couple of my favorite raw veggie pasta recipes with different sauces that are simple to make and fun to eat. If I want a Parmesan cheese substitute, I will grind up pine nuts in a food processor or Vitamix blender to get a very tasty nut version of my old favorite to sprinkle on my fresh, unprocessed pasta.

▲ ▼ ▲

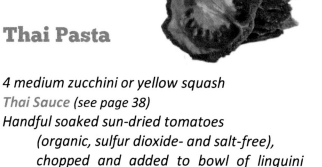

Zucchini Linguini with Marinara Sauce

See Marinara Sauce page 37

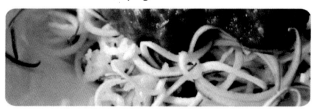

4 medium zucchini
Marinara Sauce (see page 37)

Use spiral slicer to make zucchini linguini pasta. Mix *Marinara Sauce* into the pasta and serve.

Thai Pasta

4 medium zucchini or yellow squash
Thai Sauce (see page 38)
Handful soaked sun-dried tomatoes
    (organic, sulfur dioxide- and salt-free),
    chopped and added to bowl of linguini
    pasta (optional)

Use spiral slicer to make zucchini linguini pasta. Mix *Thai Sauce* into the pasta, add chopped tomatoes (optional) and serve.

Cucumber Pasta with Orange Almond Sauce

Shared by Amanda "Lily" of
amandalily.blogspot.com

1 cucumber, spiralized
½ head red leaf lettuce, chopped into strips
1 large tomato, cubed
½ yellow bell pepper, cubed
½ cup blueberries
½ cup raspberries
Fresh herbs as desired*
1 Tablespoon raw almond butter
½ orange, juice of (about 2 Tablespoons)

Place cucumber pasta in a large bowl and top with lettuce, tomato, bell pepper, and herbs. Mix almond butter and orange juice in a small cup. Pour the sauce over the pasta just before serving. Mix well. Top with berries. Enjoy!

{ *Fresh herbs such as basil, dill, parsley, or peppermint all go well in this recipe.* }

Tip : Cubed fresh mango is a great replacement for the berries.

Raw Food Deep Dish Lasagna

Shared by Kristina Carrillo-Bucaram of
RawFullyOrganic.com and FullyRaw.com

5 large zucchinis
2 pints cherry tomatoes
Bunch Italian parsley
Bunch cilantro, arugula, spinach, each
¼ cup pine nuts (less if desired)
1 small green onion
1 small garlic clove (optional)
Marinara Sauce (see page 37)

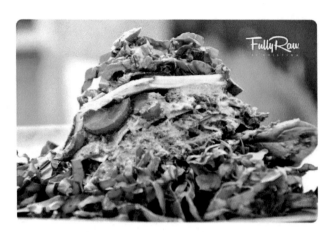

1   To make the zucchini layers, you will need a mandolin slicer or handheld mandolin. These slice the zucchini into long strips so that you can use them to separate your layers. Use about 4 zucchinis for your layers and save one for your pine nut dressing "cheese."

{ *If you want to use a few of the spinach or arugula leaves as bedding between the zucchini layers, you are welcome to do so!* }

2   After you lay your first layer into your deep dish, prepare your first layer of mixed herbs. Finely cut parsley, cilantro and spinach in a food processor. Sprinkle the herb mix on top of the zucchini shreds—"green snow!"

3   Prepare *Marinara Sauce* and spread it on top of the mixed-herb spread of the "green snow."

Tip: I did something different from just pouring my marinara onto the lasagna. I didn't want it to become watery, so I strained the marinara dressing to make it thicker. This worked fabulously! It may take some shaking with a strainer, but it will strain. Drink the yummy tomato juice afterward!

4   On top of the marinara, add another layer of zucchini strips.

5   Next, prepare second herb mix. In the food processor, cut the arugula and green onion and then sprinkle the mix on top of the zucchini.

6 Next, make "cheese" by blending one large zucchini with a small amount of pine nuts (¼ cup or less) and a clove of garlic, if you desire it for extra flavor. Spread this as the next layer in your lasagna.

I add one more layer of zucchini and then slice up my cherry tomatoes to lay them across the top.

7 Cover the cherry tomatoes with one last layer of zucchini. Press firmly as to mush everything together!

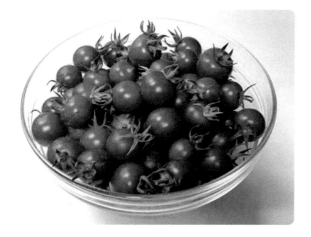

In the video I'm sharing on my YouTube channel, I finely chopped a bed of Swiss chard to place underneath the lasagna. If you want to sprinkle more marinara sauce on top, ROC IT!

My Favorite High Green Salad with Creamy Cucumber-Dill Dressing

See *Creamy Cucumber-Dill Dressing page 34*

1 Prepare the *Creamy Cucumber-Dill Dill Dressing* (see page 34)

2 The Salad Bowl: Romaine lettuce, green leaf lettuce, pea shoots, sunflower greens, chopped sweet red bell peppers and halved cherry tomatoes. Pour *Creamy Cucumber-Dill Dressing* on top of salad.

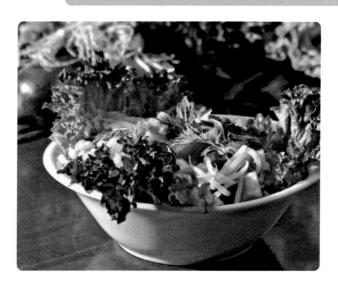

Marinated Kale Salad

1 bunch lacinato kale (also known as dinosaur kale, Tuscan kale and Italian kale)
1 avocado, cubed
1 large tomato, chopped
Juice of 1 lemon
½ cup dulse seaweed, rinsed (optional)

1 Remove the thicker part of the kale stem and slice the kale leaves chiffonade style into a bowl. Add the lemon juice and massage the kale leaves well until they wilt.

2 Add the avocado cubes and massage again. Massage to completely coat the kale leaves. Marinate for at least half an hour so the kale leaves soften. Cover with chopped tomato and dulse.

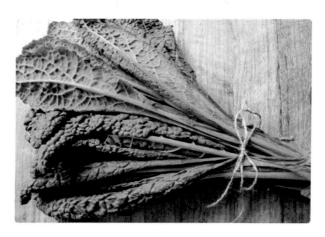

Love English Peas Salad

2 cups green peas
1 cup sunflower or clover sprouts
2 green onions, finely chopped
1 Gala apple, finely chopped
1 Tablespoon mint

Toss ingredients in a large bowl. Mix with *Creamy Avocado Dressing* (see page 35) or *Lemon Tahini Sauce* (see page 37).

Yum Avocado Mango Salad

2 mangos, peeled, seeded and chopped
1 avocado, peeled, pitted, chopped and mashed
1 handful cilantro, finely chopped

Mix all ingredients in a bowl. Add salad greens and your choice of sprouts (I love sunflower greens) around the Yum Avocado Mango Salad.

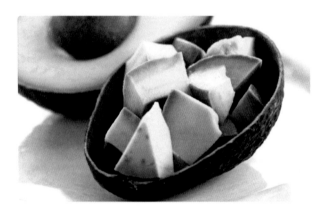

Arugula-Strawberry Salad

Shared by Lovey Jane Van Benthusen of LoveyJane.com

5-ounce bag of arugula
2 cups fresh strawberries
1 cucumber
1 ounce (small handful) soaked almonds

Blend half the strawberries and all the almonds to make a dressing. Slice the remaining strawberries and dice the cucumber, and mix it all together.

Simple, light and yummy! I love arugula!

Avocado Sprout Salad

Shared by Nomi Shannon of RawGourmet.com, author of The Raw Gourmet and other books

1-2 avocados, diced
2 cups mung bean sprouts
½ cup diced celery stalks
½ cup diced red onion (optional)
½ cup thinly sliced carrots
1 red bell pepper, diced
4 teaspoons lemon juice
2 teaspoons dulse flakes

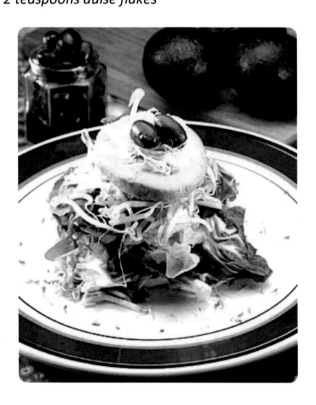

In a small bowl, combine the sprouts, celery, onion, carrots, red bell pepper, lemon juice and dulse. Toss thoroughly. Add the avocado and mix gently. Serve on lettuce leaves.

Joel's Favorite Blended Salad

Shared by Joel Brody

1 ripe tomato, chopped
3 firm celery stalks, without the leaves
6-9 leaves or more of Romaine lettuce
1 large or 2 small cucumbers,
  some of the skin scraped off
Handful or less of shelled organic raw walnuts

Place tomato into a blender or food processor first. This gives enough liquid for the blender to turn.* Add celery, lettuce, cucumber and walnuts. Blend very briefly if you want it chunkier, and for a few seconds longer if you like it smoother.

> *It can also be done without the tomato by using ½ cup of filtered water.*

Sometimes when very hungry, I simply eat the ingredients before making the recipe. I think it's preferable.

Did you know ...

The best part of raw foods, and always over 70% of them, is the <u>live water</u> they contain, filtered perfectly through their roots, vines and/or branches. I feel very strongly that the raw vegan becomes more and more intuitive while eating this way. Eventually and ideally when the tongue is clean, all fresh organic raw foods will taste utterly delicious, and recipes will become history.

Variation: *Sometimes I use additional leafy greens: fresh dill, baby spinach leaves, arugula, Napa cabbage, broccoli or cauliflower florets, etc. Sometimes, I add an organic red bell pepper. Often, I use a small avocado in place of the walnuts. Try adding fresh oregano or*

soaked and drained wakame. On rare occasions, I've also added a section of fresh turmeric.

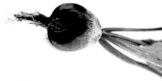

Kale-Beet-Apple Combo Delish

With *Lemon-Date Sauce, see page 36*

1 bunch kale, chopped in chiffonade slices
1 to 2 large beets, peeled and grated
1 apple, grated
Lemon-Date Sauce (see page 36).

Slice and grate the kale, beets and apple, and mix to combine. Pour the *Lemon-Date Sauce* over the mixed kale-beet-apple combo dish and combine.

Harvest Salad

Shared by Lisa Montgomery of LivingDynamically.com

All ingredients to taste:
Red beets, peeled into spirals or spiralized
Sweet potato or yams, peeled into spirals
  or spiralized
Apples, cored and diced
Peaches and/or pears, cored and diced
Raisins

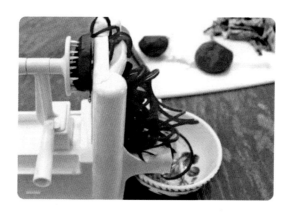

Combine all the ingredients in a bowl and serve—it is that simple.

Karen's Out-of-This-World Pineapple Coleslaw

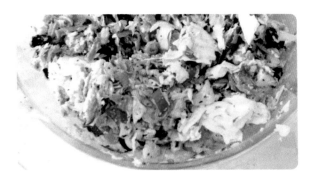

2 cups shredded green cabbage
1 cup shredded carrots
3 scallions, sliced
1 small head broccoli, shredded
4 Tablespoons finely chopped cilantro
1 cup pineapple chunks, finely chopped

For the dressing, prepare: **Lemon Tahini Sauce** *(see page 37).*

1   Shred the vegetables with a hand shredder, or in the food processor. Toss vegetables, cilantro and pineapple.

2   Prepare **Lemon Tahini Sauce**. Pour it over the coleslaw and mix.

Tabouleh

This is one of my favorite dishes. I loved it when I ate it partially cooked before I went raw in 1994, and I still love it now in 2013, but I enjoy it with ground cauliflower or sprouted quinoa instead of the old version made with bulgur wheat.

One large bunch parsley, chopped
½ large cauliflower, chopped
        or one small cauliflower
One large tomato, diced
3 scallions, diced

½ cup lemon juice
Several sprigs of mint
One avocado, diced (optional)

1   Process cauliflower in the food processor with the S blade until well ground. Remove the cauliflower from the food processor and place in a large bowl.

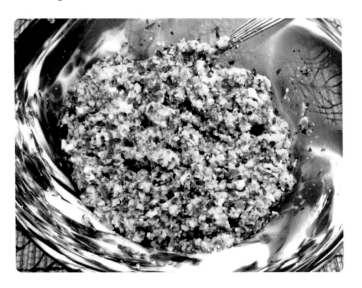

2   Then food process parsley, tomato, scallions, lemon juice and mint*. Pulse several times until well mixed. Add optional diced avocado last, and mix thoroughly.

Variation: *Diced cucumber could also be added afterward for variation.*

Romaine Burritos

One head of large Romaine lettuce leaves

For Taco Filling:
1 cup almonds or walnuts, presoaked 8-12 hours
½ cup lemon juice
¼ cup sun-dried tomatoes,*
        presoaked 2 hours, chopped
2 scallions, finely chopped
1 teaspoon each: ground cumin, coriander
        and paprika (¼ cup fresh cilantro can be
substituted for the ground coriander)

1   Put all ingredients into a food processor with an "S" blade. Process until smooth, or until the consistency of a traditional bean dip. Add a little water if needed to get it moving.

2   Spread taco filling on the lettuce leaves. Top with fresh *Tomato Salsa* (see page 37) or *Tormatilo Sauce* (see page 36) for an extra taste sensation.

> *Salt-free, organic sun-dried tomatoes. The conventional variety of sun-dried tomatoes is treated with sulfur dioxide to keep a bright red color and also contains dangerous amounts of salt.*

Cauliflower Spanish Rice

1 head of cauliflower
2 to 3 Tablespoons scallions, chopped
¼ cup fresh cilantro, chopped
1 cup sun-dried tomatoes, soaked and chopped
1 avocado
Juice of 1 lime
1 teaspoon cumin
1 red bell pepper, finely chopped
1 large tomato, finely chopped

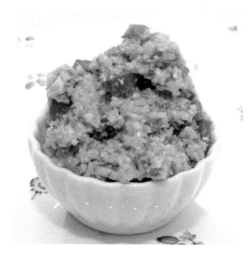

1   Cut cauliflower into pieces and chop to a rice texture in a food processor. Place chopped cauliflower in a large serving bowl.

2   In the food processor pulse scallion and cilantro and then add to the bowl of cauliflower.

3   Chop avocado into the food processor, add sun-dried tomatoes, lime juice and cumin and process until smooth.

4   Combine avocado mixture with cauliflower rice. Add red bell pepper and tomato and mix all ingredients together one last time.

Nori Rolls with Carrot-Ginger Dip

See *Carrot-Ginger Dip* page 41

Untoasted nori sheets
Raw nut or seed butter, nut or seed pâté
or half an avocado (see Dips and Pâtés recipes, page 40-41)
1 lettuce, shredded
1 cucumber julienne
1 tomato, chopped
Sprouts (we like clover sprouts and sunflower greens)

Variation: Add shredded carrots, red bell pepper strips and soaked sun-dried tomatoes.

There are numerous ways to make delicious nori rolls. On busy days, we would just place a thin strip of raw nut butter or we'd mash half of an avocado on the raw nori sheets, add lettuce, cucumber julienne, chopped tomatoes, and sprouts, and roll them up.

> *Rub a lemon half on the edges of the sheet to seal the roll.*

Wraps like this are a fun way to serve food, and kids love them. Large lettuce or cabbage leaves also make wonderful wraps filled with lots of veggies mixed with some mashed avocado or a spread of nut or seed butter or pâté.

Tip: *Try the **Root Veggies Pâté** (see page 41) with some shredded green leafy vegetables inside a wrap. Yum!*

Sushi

Shared by Anna Chmielewska of SweetVeganNature.com

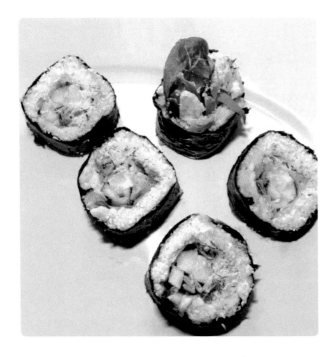

1 large cauliflower, shredded in
    food   processor into rice size
Carrots, grated or julienned
1 avocado, sliced
1 cucumber, cut lengthwise into square strips
Lettuce leaves
Raw sesame seeds (optional)
Untoasted nori sheets
Spread of choice (see recipes page 40-41)

1   Lay a nori sheet on rolling mat (or directly on cutting board), shiny side down.

2   Spread 1 cup of the cauliflower "rice" over the nori sheet using wet hands, leaving at least a ½-inch strip of nori uncovered at the bottom.

3   Place lettuce first followed by the spread of choice, carrots, avocado and cucumber. Sprinkle with sesame seeds.

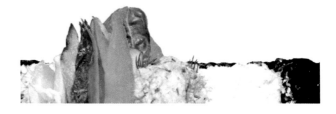

4   Using rolling mat or just hands, begin to tightly roll sushi. Start at the side nearest you and roll away from you. Moisten ending edge with wet hands to "glue" nori sheet. When sushi is completely rolled, use rolling mat or hands to gently squeeze sushi so it doesn't unroll when cutting.

5   Using very sharp knife to produce clean cut, slice sushi into 6 or 8 pieces, depending on desired thickness.

Tip 1: *It helps to wet the knife before cutting the sushi so the fillings won't stick to it.*

Tip 2: *Serve with **Tahini Sauce**: mix tahini with lemon juice and finely grated ginger.*

Guacamole Wraps

Best to eat along with a large salad.

2 small ripe avocados
1 large tomato, diced
2 or more Tablespoons fresh cilantro,
    chopped
½ teaspoon ground cumin (optional)
2 Tablespoons fresh lime or lemon juice
1 large head of Romaine lettuce leaves

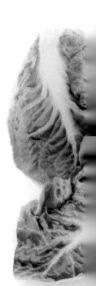

1   Mash the avocados. Add cilantro, cumin and lime or lemon juice. Top with diced tomatoes, or a raw salsa.

2   Fill each Romaine leaf with the guacamole mixture, roll it up and place a toothpick through it to keep it closed until ready to eat.

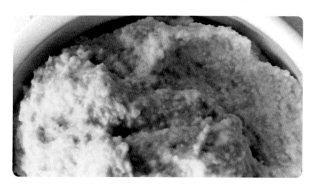

Variation: Try with soaked sun-dried tomatoes and sprouts, especially sunflower sprouts.

Good Ole Collards and Sweet Peppers

An adaptation of a recipe from the book Raw Foods on A Budget *by Brandi Rollins of RawFoodsOnABudget.com*

4 medium collard green leaves
Juice from ½ lemon
14 Brazil nuts
1 medium sweet red bell pepper, diced

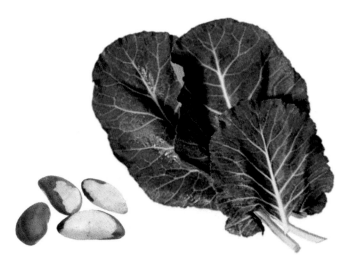

1   Layer the collard leaves on top of each other, roll them into a burrito and cut them into thin ¼-inch slices. Place the sliced collards into a large bowl and add the lemon juice and mix well. Add diced sweet bell peppers.

2   Grind Brazil nuts into flour, using a coffee grinder, food processor, or high-speed blender. Sprinkle the nut flour over the greens, and mix until the greens are well coated, leaving 2-3 tablespoons to sprinkle on top of the dish before serving. Enjoy!

Brandi's Collard Salad can be a light side salad or placed on top of a plate of mixed leafy greens to create a full meal. I've made this recipe and love it most in the fall and winter, when collards are in season.

Chili

Shared by Dr. Timothy Trader

8 organic tomatoes, diced
1 medium zucchini, diced
8 organic sun-dried tomatoes
4 medium organic red bell peppers, diced
1 packed cup sweet tamarind,
     shells removed and deseeded
2 Tablespoons organic raw tahini (optional)*

You can find tamarind at an Asian or Mexican grocery. The tamarind will make a difference for the kids and others to enjoy these recipes. Tamarind also makes for good food combining, as it makes a far better combination with acid foods than, say, dates.

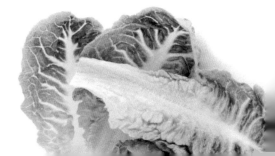

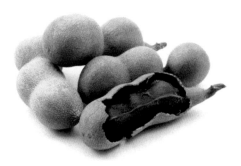

Blend 3 of the tomatoes and 3 of the red bell peppers with all of the zucchini and tamarind. When creamy, pour over the remaining diced tomatoes and red bell peppers, and mix thoroughly. Serves two for a main dinner entrée.

Variation: Optional tahini can add some zest and thickness to the blend.

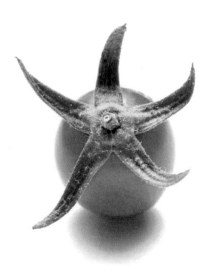

Gail's Veggie Burger

Shared by Gail Zikri of NewEarthKitchen.com

Dehydration time: *1-2 hours, optional*

½ cup sunflower seeds—soaked overnight
    and rinsed in the morning
½ cup macadamia nuts
¼ red bell pepper
1 zucchini
¼ small red onion

½ cup mushrooms
¼ bunch of cilantro or parsley, minced
½ teaspoon of your favorite herbs, fresh or dried

1   Place the sprouted sunflower seeds, nuts and seasoning in food processor and mix together. Do not over mix–leave it a little chunky. Place into a mixing bowl.

2   In food processor, mince the red bell pepper, red onion, cilantro or parsley, zucchini and mushroom. Add to the mixing bowl and mix well. Add herbs to taste.

{ If mixture is too dry or heavy, add a little more vegetables or some water. }

3   Use hands to form 'patty-like' shapes, between 1½-2½ inches and place them on the Teflex sheet on dehydrator tray.

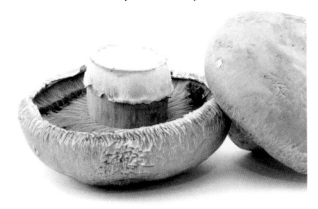

4   Ready to serve, or dehydrate at 105 degrees for 3 hours, or until a little crispy on the outside. Halfway through, turn patties over and remove Teflex sheet. Do not over dehydrate—they should be a little moist inside.

Storage: Cover tightly and refrigerate leftovers. Will last up to 3 days in a fridge. Can be frozen for up to 1 month. Serve any time. Goes well with any green salad, coleslaw, savory soupor veggies.

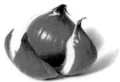

Bok Choy Stew

Shared by Chris Kendall of TheRawAdvantage.com

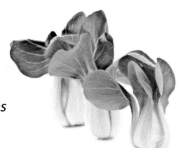

1½ pounds bok choy
5 tomatoes
1 mango
1 medium zucchini
¼ cup sun-dried tomatoes
1 bunch cilantro

1   Chop the zucchini into cubes, roughly chop half of the tomatoes and stems of bok choy and put in a bowl, placing bok choy greens aside.

2   Blend remaining tomatoes with mango, bok choy greens, cilantro and sun-dried tomatoes. Mix all together and enjoy one of my favorites!

Italian Pumpkin Seed

Shared by Chris Kendall of TheRawAdvantage.com

3 Tablespoons raw pumpkin seeds
10 tomatoes
¼ cup sun-dried tomatoes
1 bunch basil
1 lime

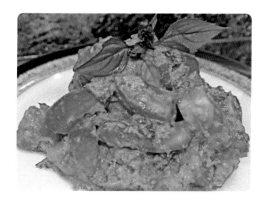

1   Cut top ¼ off all tomatoes and blend with juice of lime, ⅓ of sun-dried tomatoes and ⅔ of pumpkin seeds.

2   Dice the remaining tomatoes, chop basil and mix well with dressing.

3   Add remaining pumpkin seeds and sun-dried tomatoes. Pour over the top, and enjoy this creamy classic!

Faux Bolognese

Shared by Chris Kendall of TheRawAdvantage.com

¼ cauliflower
2 medium zucchini
4 tomatoes
½-1 mango
¼ cup sun-dried tomatoes
Basil and oregano to taste

1   Using chosen method, make zucchini noodles of desired thickness and shape (I prefer making thin, angel -hair noodles). Save zucchini bits for later.

2   Squeeze juice from tomatoes (drink, or use in a salad dressing) and blend with mango, sun-dried tomatoes and herbs.

3   Add the cauliflower and any zucchini bits, pulsing sauce until desired chunkiness.

Variation: Use 1 Medjool date instead of mango. Add 1 green onion for a more "traditionally" flavored sauce.

Zuccanoes

Shared by Julia Lucas of RawJulia.com
Dehydration time: 6-7 hours

2 medium zucchinis
¼ cup raw acorn or butternut squash, cubed
¼ cup red bell pepper
½ cup of sunflower seeds or walnuts, presoaked
Juice of ½ lemon

1 small clove of garlic (optional)
½ teaspoon fresh rosemary
½ cup kale, spinach or other greens

1   Cut zucchinis in half lengthwise and spoon out some of the zucchini seeds to create "canoes."

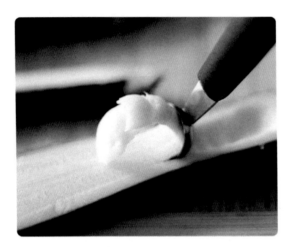

2   Place the zucchini seeds and all the other ingredients in a blender. Blend until well-combined. Mixture should be kind of chunky. If some greens make the mixture too soupy, add more nuts or seeds.

3   Fill the "canoes" with prepared mix.

4   Dehydrate on mesh trays at 105 degrees for 6-7 hours.

This recipe can be played with to accommodate your taste and adjusted to what you have in the cupboard.

Live Veggie and Fruit Kabobs
with fresh *Tomato Marinade* (see page 37)

*Live Veggie and Fruit Kabobs are especially fun in the summertime, placed on skewers. The usual barbecued fare is toxic, especially because it contains **acrylamide**. This recipe makes a healthful live replacement.*

Cherry tomatoes
Red bell peppers
Cauliflower
Broccoli
Zucchini
Mushrooms
Tomato Marinade (see page 37)

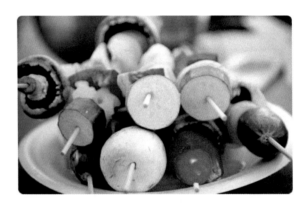

1   Chop vegetables and fruits into large pieces and leave to marinate all in a *Tomato Marinade* for a few hours.

2   Place veggies on metal or wooden skewers and dehydrate for several hours until slightly softened.

Orange Glad-to-Eat-Me Meal

Shared by Windsor Griffing, age 16, of RawFoodCentral.com

5 oranges, pulsed in processor till chunky
2 cups whole blueberries
15 almonds, powdered in high-speed blender

Place oranges in a bowl and place blueberries on top. Sprinkle with the powdered almonds on top of the mixture. Enjoy!

Party Food

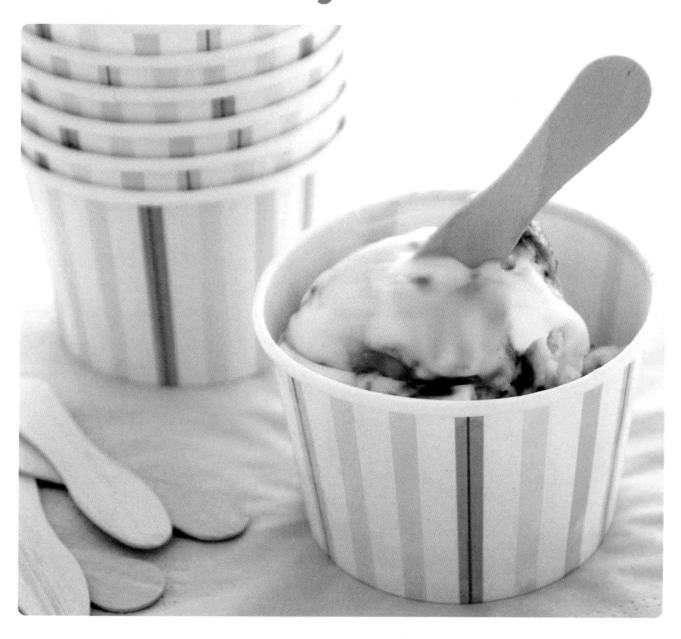

Banana Fun Pops

This is a favorite at holiday time and parties.

¼ cup pine nuts
5 bananas
Water to process

1   Chop nuts in the food processor, add bananas and continue until smooth. Add a little water if needed.

2   Pour into paper Dixie cups and freeze. After an hour, place a wooden craft stick into the middle of each pop. Freeze for at least 5 hours.

Simple Raw Vegan Blueberry Pie

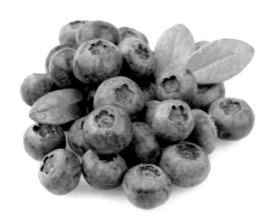

5-6 bananas, sliced
1 pint fresh blueberries
7-10 soaked dates
Dried shredded coconut

1   Line a 9-inch pie plate with banana slices.

2   Blend blueberries with soaked dates and pour the mixture over the sliced bananas.

3   Decorate the top with sprinkles of dried shredded coconut. Chill for two hours in the refrigerator until it jells from the natural pectin in the blueberries—a big success at get-togethers and parties.

Watch my YouTube video on creating this simple and delicious potluck favorite pie: YouTube.com/watch?v=Nv9EYzIN_dg

My Favorite Quick Apple Pie

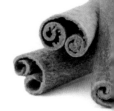

Crust:
1 cup of soaked pecans, drained
1 cup of shredded coconut
10 dates, soaked until soft enough for processing

Process in food processor until smooth and well mixed. Place in a glass pie plate and spread to cover. If time permits, let it set in a refrigerator for a few hours.

Filling:
4 apples, cored and chopped
     in the food processor with peels
¾ teaspoon cinnamon
2½ teaspoons lemon juice

Spread the filling over the crust. Top with thin banana, apple, pear, or kiwi slices, or with blueberries. The fruit covering makes the pie festive for the holidays.

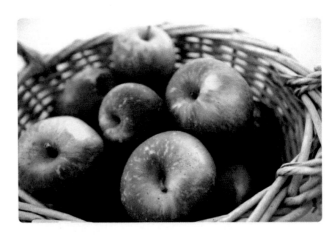

Berry Good Pie

Shared by Dr. Douglas Graham of
FoodNSport.com

10 ounces frozen strawberries
12 ounces blueberries
8 ounces blackberries
4 ounces raspberries
4 ounces young coconut meat
6 ounces young coconut milk
6 ounces very ripe pineapple

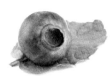

1   Use a Champion juicer with the blank plate. Mix enough frozen strawberries to make a "crust." Add a layer of blueberries and a layer of blackberries. Top with a layer of thinly sliced strawberries.

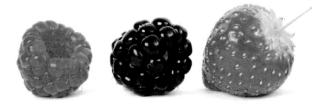

2   Blend coconut milk and meat with pineapple, and pour over pie dish until it is full. Decorate with a ring of raspberries. Freeze and serve.

Orange-"Choco"-Banana Pie

Shared by Anna Chmielewska of
SweetVeganNature.com

Crust:
1 cup of dates
½ cup dried, unsweetened shredded coconut
lemon or lime zest from 1 lemon (optional)

Mix all ingredients in a food processor until well-combined and sticky. Transport the crust batter onto a small cake pan and form a nice even bottom. Use wet hands to distribute the crust easily.

Chocolate cream:
2 bananas
2 Medjool dates
2 Tablespoons carob
½ teaspoon vanilla extract (optional)
Small pinch chili powder (optional)

Orange cream:
2 oranges, peeled
1 Tablespoon chia seeds
1 slice lemon, peeled
Zest from 1 lemon and 1 orange

Filling:
2 bananas, sliced

Creams: Mix ingredients in a food processor until creamy (process creams separately). Let the orange cream sit for 15 minutes for the chia seeds to expand.

1   Place a layer of chocolate cream on crust and cover with banana slices. Leave ¼ of the cream for finish.

2   Spread the orange cream on top and cover with banana slices. Finish with a thin ring of the remaining chocolate cream around the edge.

3   Freeze 2-3 hours before serving.

{ *The pie can be prepared days before planned serving. Store the pie in the freezer.* }

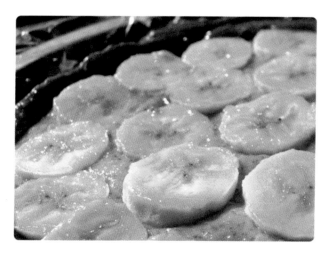

"Love" Raspberry Pie

Shared by Anna Chmielewska of
SweetVeganNature.com

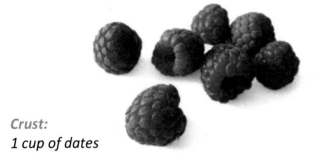

Crust:
1 cup of dates

Chop dates in a food processor until a sticky paste. Use wet hands to distribute the date paste onto a cake pan and form even crust bottom. Use 3- to 4-inch-wide round cake pan.*

Filling:
2 bananas, frozen
2 cups raspberries
3 Medjool dates
1 Tablespoon lemon juice

Mix all ingredients in the food processor until creamy and smooth. Pour the cream onto the date crust and enjoy or refrigerate before serving.

{ *Use a heart-shaped cake pan or a cookie cutter on the plate, to make your perfect "Love" Pie!* }

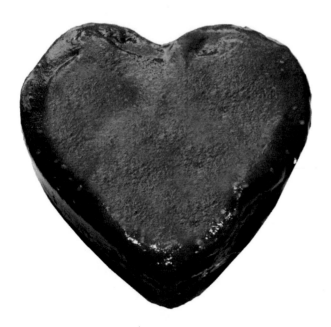

Strawberry Tart

Shared by Amanda "Lily" of
amandalily.blogspot.com

1 cup shredded coconut
8 Medjool dates
*2 cups organic strawberries, sliced**

1   Place coconut and dates in a food processor and process until mixed and starting to clump.

2   Divide crust mixture among 6 lined muffin tin cups. Press down and then up the sides to form crust.

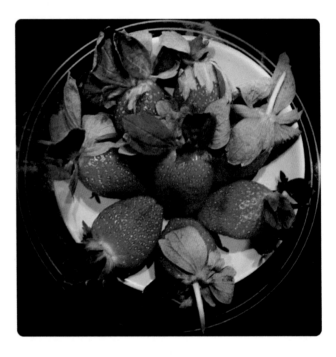

3   Place strawberries in the food processor. Pulse until they are chopped into small pieces and just starting to release their juice.

4   Divide filling into six crusts and press down with a tablespoon.

5   Place tarts in a fridge for at least an hour so they can set before serving.

{ *Strawberries must be organic for the tarts to be flavorful.* }

Ice Cream Variations

Plain banana ice cream is made with frozen bananas placed through the Champion juicer with the blank plate in. As an alternative, use a food processor, but you will need to add a little water to process.

There are many variations you can create by mixing bananas with other frozen fruit and/or carob.*

Variations: Make ice cream from frozen bananas with any of these frozen fruits:

- *mangos*
- *peaches*
- *strawberries*
- *pineapple*

or carob for healthy choco-banana ice cream.

Did you know ...

Carob is a delicious fruit with a similar taste and color to chocolate, but it doesn't contain any caffeine or theobromine. According to Wikipedia, "The carob tree, Ceratonia siliqua, is a leguminous evergreen shrub or tree of the family Leguminosae (pulse family) native to the Mediterranean region. It is cultivated for its edible seedpods. Carobs are also known as St. John's bread. According to tradition of some Christians, St. John the Baptist subsisted on them in the wilderness. A similar legend exists of Rabbi Shimon bar Yochai and his son."

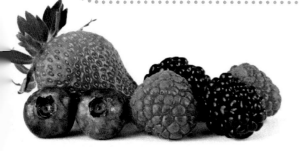

I keep frozen fruits in covered glass dishes in the freezer. I used to freeze the fruits in plastic bags, but research has shown dioxins from the plastic can be released into the food, especially during freezing or heating.

Ice Cream

Shared by Margrieta Lasmane

4 frozen bananas
5 Medjool dates
1 Tablespoon carob powder
One orange or mango for better food combining

Blend all ingredients and enjoy a fantastic raw ice cream.

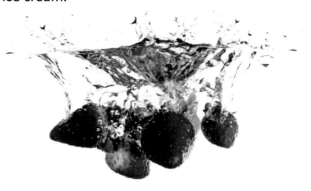

Banana-Mango-Strawberry Ice Cream

5 bananas, frozen in a glass dish to avoid toxins
  from plastic containers
1 cup mango flesh, frozen in a glass dish
1 cup strawberries, frozen
½ teaspoon vanilla powder (optional)
Water as needed

1   Freeze fruit overnight.

2   Process frozen fruit one at a time in a food processor or blend in a Vitamix until smooth and creamy. Place each in its own bowl.

3   Make colorful dishes by first placing banana, then mango, and then strawberry ice cream, one on top of the other. Add vanilla powder if desired.

Banana Splits with Strawberry Sauce

2 bananas, sliced lengthwise
1 cup fresh strawberries

1   Slice bananas lengthwise and place them on a plate facing up.

2   Blend one cup of fresh strawberries to the consistency of syrup, and pour over the open-face bananas.

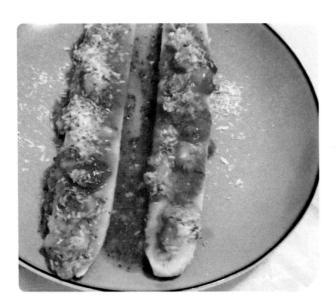

Variations: *Three Medjool dates may be added to the strawberry blend for a thicker consistency. Other treats, such as shredded coconut, may be added as a topping*

Mango-Coconut-Mint "Ice Cream"

Shared from "DESSERT: Making It Rich Without Oil" by Dr. Ritamarie Loscalzo and Chef Karen Osborne of drritamarie.com/makeitrich/

½ cup coconut water,
      from a young Thai coconut
¼ cup coconut meat, from a young Thai coconut
2 pitted Medjool dates
10 ounces frozen mango
1 Tablespoon of fresh peppermint leaves
      or 1 teaspoon of dried peppermint leaves

1   Blend the coconut water, coconut meat and dates in a high-speed blender until smooth.

2   Add the mint and frozen mango and blend again until smooth. Enjoy!

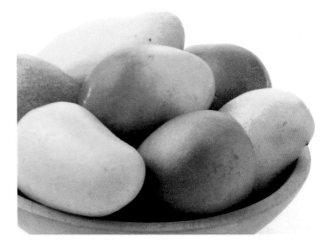

Superfood Peppermint Thins

Shared from DESSERT: Making It Rich Without Oil by Dr. Ritamarie Loscalzo and Chef Karen Osborne of DrRitaMarie.com/MakeItRich/

These treats are much better for you than the peppermint patties you may have eaten before.

½ cup hemp seeds
1 cup finely shredded unsweetened
    dried coconut
¼ teaspoon green stevia powder
4 drops peppermint essential oil
1 teaspoon chlorella powder
1/8 teaspoon ground vanilla beans
    or vanilla extract
1/8 cup Brazil nuts

Process all the ingredients in a food processor until almost smooth. Spread the mixture thin on a tray lined with wax or parchment paper, and score into desired sizes. Freeze for at least half an hour.

Tip: *To score, make shallow cuts in the surface of the batter so that it will easily break apart into the desired size and shape when dry. It works best to press down through the mixture with a pizza rocker, but a knife can be used as well.*

Cheezy Kale Chips

Dehydration time 6-plus hours

1 large bunch kale, de-stemmed
    and leaves torn off
½ cup raw macadamia nuts, soaked for 2 hours
1 cup red bell pepper, chopped
1 small zucchini, chopped
2 Tablespoons lemon or lime juice
1 teaspoon curry powder
½ teaspoon dulse flakes

1   Place kale in a large bowl.

2   Mix red bell pepper with lemon or lime juice in a high speed blender until smooth. Add macadamia nuts and blend (additional water may be necessary to move the nuts in the blender). Add zucchini, curry powder, and dulse flakes and blend until smooth but thick. Pour over kale pieces and coat well.

3   Place kale pieces on nonstick Teflex sheets on top of dehydrator trays and dehydrate 6 or more hours at 110 degrees until dry. Kale should be rotated to dry throughout.

Green Kabobs

Shared by Brian Rossiter of Fruit-Powered.com

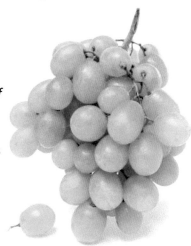

1 pound of green grapes
6 kiwis
1 cucumber
3 stalks of celery
1 lemon

Split the cucumber in half and scoop out the seeds, and peel the cucumber if desired. Slice the kiwis, cucumber halves and celery stalks into bite-size chunks. Add to skewers with grapes. If desired, drizzle the juice of a lemon over the Green Kabobs.

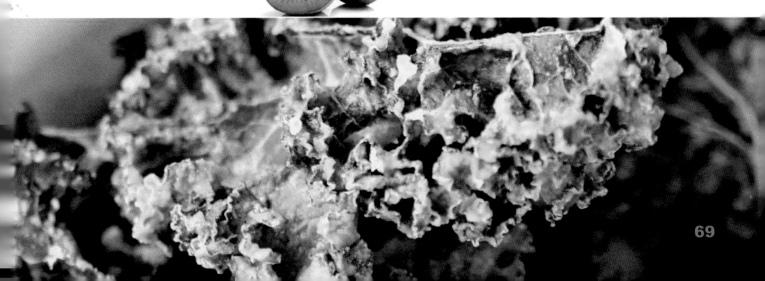

Additional Reading

Try some of my tips to help kids love eating leafy green vegetables, discover natural home remedies, get information on the best ways for parents to detoxify, and learn how best to use nuts and seeds, all for a healthy and happy lifestyle.

Knowledge of healthy eating principles is fundamental so start with understanding food-combining basics.

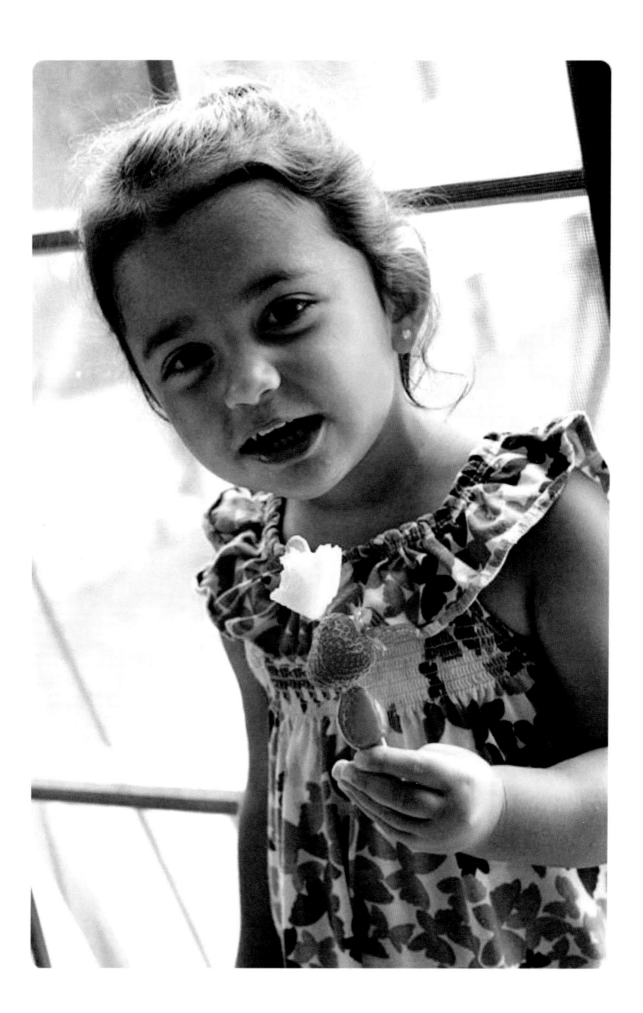

Food-Combining Chart

Food Combining Chart

DO NOT EAT FRUIT WITH ANY OTHER FOOD EXCEPT GREEN NON-STARCHY VEGETABLES

ACID FRUIT		SUB-ACID FRUIT		SWEET FRUIT	MELON	
Blackberries	Pineapple	Apple	Kiwi	Bananas	Cantaloupe	Honey Dew
Grapefruit	Raspberries	Apricot	Mango	Dates	Casaba	Persian
Lemon	Strawberries	Blueberries	Nectarine	Dried Fruit	Crane	Sharlyn
Lime	Tangerines	Cherimoya	Papaya	Thompson &	Crenshaw	Watermelon
Orange	Tomatoes[1]	Cherries	Peach	Muscat Grapes		
		Fresh Fig	Pear	Persimmon	[Eat before other fruits]	
[Eat before other fruits]		Grapes	Plums	Raisins		

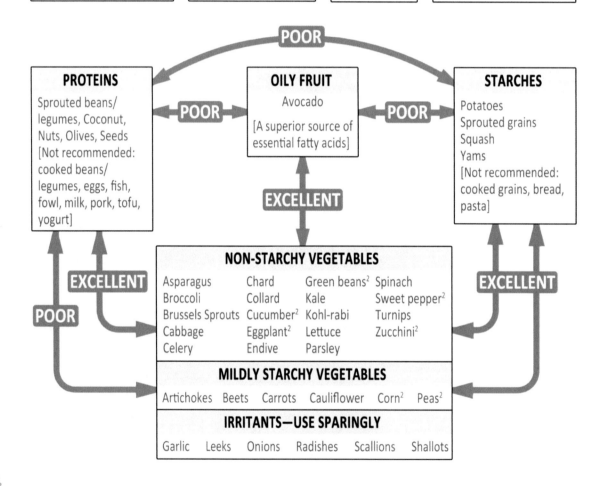

PROTEINS
Sprouted beans/
legumes, Coconut,
Nuts, Olives, Seeds
[Not recommended:
cooked beans/
legumes, eggs, fish,
fowl, milk, pork, tofu,
yogurt]

OILY FRUIT
Avocado
[A superior source of
essential fatty acids]

STARCHES
Potatoes
Sprouted grains
Squash
Yams
[Not recommended:
cooked grains, bread,
pasta]

POOR — EXCELLENT — POOR

EXCELLENT

NON-STARCHY VEGETABLES

Asparagus	Chard	Green beans[2]	Spinach
Broccoli	Collard	Kale	Sweet pepper[2]
Brussels Sprouts	Cucumber[2]	Kohl-rabi	Turnips
Cabbage	Eggplant[2]	Lettuce	Zucchini[2]
Celery	Endive	Parsley	

MILDLY STARCHY VEGETABLES

Artichokes   Beets   Carrots   Cauliflower   Corn[2]   Peas[2]

IRRITANTS—USE SPARINGLY

Garlic   Leeks   Onions   Radishes   Scallions   Shallots

[1] Tomatoes only combine with non-starchy vegetables, seeds, nuts, olives, avocados, cucumbers and sweet peppers.
[2] Botanically classified as a fruit, but its bio-chemical composition places it in a non-fruit food combining category.

Source: David Klein, Ph.D., Colitis & Crohn's Health Recovery Center, **Colitis-Crohns.com**
and **DigestionPerfection.com**

Fast-Food Advertising at Sports Events

I recently attended a professional baseball game at a large stadium. I hadn't been to a game for many years and was horrified to see fast food offered at every stand. Hamburgers, hot dogs, pizza, meatballs, French fries, pretzels, Cracker Jack, cotton candy, soft drinks, beer and other fast foods abounded everywhere.

When I was growing up in the 1950s and '60s, I remember eating French fries that were served in a small white paper pocket. Neither my friends nor I made a whole meal of French fries. On this day at the baseball game, I saw people eating huge portions of French fries served on large plates. A very important Swedish nutritional study completed at the University of Stockholm, reveals when starches, such as in French fries, form a golden-brown crust after being heated at high temperatures, they undergo a chemical reaction forming a carcinogenic plastic called acrylamide. Chips contain even greater percentages of acrylamide.

Wikipedia states, "Advertising campaigns for fast- food restaurants have changed in their intent over time. Many modern campaigns stress the availability of healthy options after years of criticism for the harmful effects of a fast-food diet. The rise in awareness of healthy eating and obesity has negatively impacted the business of these establishments, and their marketing campaigns have attempted to rectify this." From what I saw while walking around the stadium, this did not seem to be a reality. There was no mention of any nutrient-dense fruits or vegetables anywhere. The obesity rate in that one venue was alarmingly high. Animal-based, processed and refined foods served at the stands were advertised repeatedly on the large, centrally placed stadium screen. It was easy to see that the meat and dairy council as well as processed food distributors have a large monopoly over what gets sold at sports events. You would want to think that good forms of exercise should coincide with the healthful foods that create healthy bodies. Fruit consumption is known to enhance athletic capability and performance, but fruits were nowhere to be found.

Unfortunately for today's children, most fast-food chains target their advertising at children and teenagers from whom they make a large percentage of their profits. I still recall the many years of beef jerky, doughnut holes and potato chips served at my children's weekly soccer and baseball games. There were the occasional orange slices, but these weren't viewed as the fun snacks. Once I brought a big bowl of fresh organic strawberries for the end-of-game snack, and the children devoured them, but that didn't lead to other parents' bringing the same kind of healthful fare when it was their turn to bring snacks.

As the benefits of a raw food lifestyle become more widely recognized, let's hope the public at large will understand that fruits and vegetables are the best foods to provide energy, stamina and lasting health.

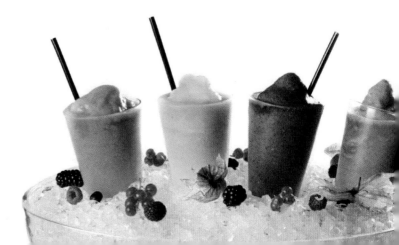

9 Tips to Get Children to Eat Their Fruits and Vegetables

In this article, I would like to share some of the many creative tips I've learned along the way to encourage children to eat more fruits and vegetables.

1   Try different textures. For example, a child may not like leafy green vegetables in a salad but may enjoy them in green smoothies, juices, soups or dips.

2   Keep fruits and vegetables around the kitchen in pretty baskets and brightly colored bowls. Children will find the varied colors of the foods in their everyday environment attractive.

3   Give the foods you make lively or catchy names. My kids created their own recipes, even from the time they were very little, and they gave them names. For example, BAT (banana, apple and a scoop of tahini) was a cereal that worked very well for replacing the processed packaged cereals, and it became a family favorite.

4   Kids love using equipment. A spiral slicer for making veggie pasta; a snow cone maker for making ices from fresh fruit juice for a special birthday party treat; a small juicer (such as The Healthy Juicer); a mini food processor; the Champion Juicer for making all sorts of recipes, especially banana ice cream; and a dehydrator for making crackers, veggie burgers and veggie chips at low temperatures to preserve the quality of the food.

5   Play "Health Food Restaurant"–let your kids be the chefs! Your children will love setting up counters and preparing smoothies, juices, fruit or veggie platters, guacamole, coleslaw, wraps, and beautiful salads. My children often used a doorway as their ideal place to set up their restaurant. Ironing board or a small table was the counter. Even when we traveled, we bought food for them to prepare meals for us in our hotel room, and my husband and I would be the customers, paying them for our meals!

6   Kids love dips! I observe so many children eating their leafy greens (such as kale, Romaine lettuce and spinach) and other veggies while delighting in home-made dips made from fruits, vegetables and herbs, such as basil, cilantro (coriander) or dill, as well as nuts and seeds.

7   Kids adore attractive food designs that create a picture. For example, a half-inch-thick pineapple circle can be used to make the "sun" and a bowl of orange sections makes the "sun's rays." I've used a heart-shaped stainless steel cake pan to prepare special raw treats for Valentine's Day. I bought different ridge-edged cutters to make decorative trims on cucumbers, cantaloupes, peppers and carrots. Children like appealing and fun designs in food, so why not use these tools for making fun shapes with raw foods? It's also easy to find many different cookie-cutter shapes and holiday designs for making cookies, cakes and other treats.

8   Use of puppetry with young children is an excellent way to introduce them to fresh, unprocessed fruits and vegetables and playfully encourage discussion of healthful living topics.

9   Traveling with your children provides an excellent learning experience and creates family bonding time. We were always able to find fruits and vegetables during our travels to Costa Rica, Colombia, Switzerland and Italy. It was exciting to look up and identify specific fruits or vegetables in the book, *Fruits and Vegetables of the World,* by Michel Viard, and then locate them in markets at each new destination.

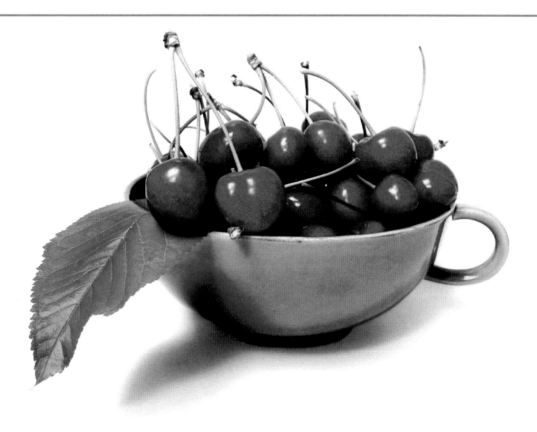

5 Tips for Getting Your Kids to Eat Their Leafy Greens

I teach a bi-annual class titled "Raw Food Fun for Families," a fun, lively workshop to provide children and their parents with a supportive framework for incorporating more fresh raw foods into their lifestyle. Every class includes parents who are frustrated with their spouse and/or children who have an aversion to leafy green vegetables. So I came up with 5 tips to help kids learn to enjoy those nutrient-dense, green-colored friends from the plant kingdom.

1   Change the texture. For example, a child may not like leafy green vegetables in salads but may love them in green juices, green smoothies, green soups, green puddings, green dips, or green dressings. My son will eat leafy green salads, jazzed up with shredded carrots, sliced tomatoes, and chopped radishes, but will not go near green smoothies or soups.

2   Make the leafy greens part of an attractive design. Encourage your kids to create artwork with their leafy green veggies. Ask them to put together a leafy green collage. When complete, the family gets to sample it together!

3   Kids love dips! Add healthy, delicious fresh herbs and it's even more likely they'll dip their dark green lettuces, kale, celery, spinach or other leafy greens. If they have something really yummy into which to dip their fresh leafy greens, they'll be more likely to indulge. Favorite dips for us included those made from raw tahini (sesame seed paste) and Creamy Cucumber-Dill (Dill is so refreshing—my daughter has always loved any dressing that is livened up with dill). Most children will be attracted to one or more of the fresh green herbs: parsley, dill, cilantro, basil, etc. Adding one of these to a new dip recipe could be the key to dipping those leafy greens! (My son adores parsley, and so I'll add loads of it to a Tabouleh recipe).

4   Get your kids hungry, and there's a good chance they'll eat leafy green vegetables. When we would take rides, as on field trips, I would bring some leafy green vegetables along with something more filling such as pâtés, or homemade nut butters. This was the perfect time for them to enjoy the green leaves. Especially when used as a wrap, they ate significant amounts of those wonderful greens!

5   Getting your child to work in the garden will most likely be the most important of these tips. Harvesting your blooming crops together as a family will provide the profound connection to all that is Nature, and the sampling of Earth's bounty will speak to the child about the natural food for humans.

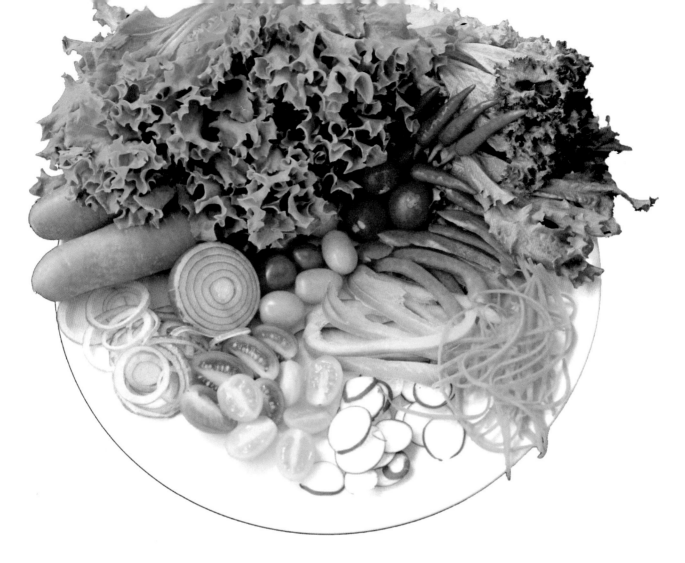

Getting your children to love their leafy green vegetables can be a daunting task, but once they're hooked, it's usually for life. The family and peer support in my class "Raw Food Fun for Families" brings leafy green vegetables to life in many simple recipes. We all need to create this same fun environment in our homes.

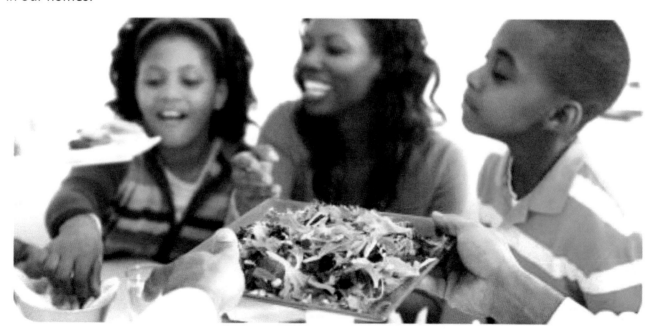

10 Tips to Bring Relaxation and Calm into Your Family Life During the Holidays

1 Exercise daily. Moving your body burns up stress hormones, leaving you relaxed and refreshed.

2 Seek support in your life by reaching out to others. Get the help you need, especially at holiday time, when daily life can be more stressful.

3 Eat an abundance of nutrient-dense raw vegan foods to energize and keep spirits up.

4 Get adequate sleep to feel more relaxed. When overwhelmed with chores and shopping to do, this is most important.

5 Breathe deeply. Inhale slowly, letting your stomach rise for five seconds. Hold, and exhale slowly for five seconds. Practice five times each day for a total of five minutes.

6 Practice acceptance. "Accepting whatever you cannot change" will provide a peaceful feeling in dealing with the world.

7 A loving atmosphere in your home is the foundation of your life. When you and your loved ones have a disagreement, focus only on the current situation. Do not bring up the past.

8 Pleasing melodies, especially Mozart, have great value for the entire family, a form of meditation that calms as well as uplifts the spirit.

9 Meditate. Sitting in quiet meditation even for 15 minutes a day will create a more focused and rested mind. Silence creates an avenue for dealing with all life's situations.

10 Have fun! Make sure the preparations and stress that come along with the holidays don't affect your family life. The well-being of each individual is a more important focus than the preparations involved for a beautiful holiday table. If the preparations are easy and fun, then even the youngest child will want to be involved.

Natural Home Remedies for the Health-Conscious Family

*M*any natural home remedies can be used for a variety of ailments without resorting to toxic over-the-counter drugs.

Children's colds are usually accompanied by a fever of 100 to 101 degrees, little or no appetite, fussiness, sore throat and/or cough, and runny nose. Other possible complications such as middle-ear infections may also be present.

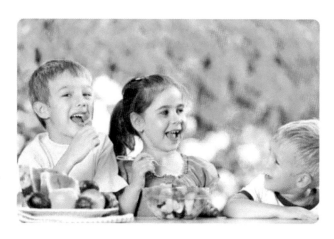

The most common cause of colds in children is a **mucus-forming diet** and unhealthful lifestyle choices. Always look at the diet first when a child is experiencing frequent colds. Any milk products, raw or pasteurized, are mucus-forming and cold-producing. Unprocessed fruits and vegetables should make up a large part of the diet. Young children especially cannot digest processed foods, resulting in undigested food particles that compromise their immunity. When parents serve as models for healthful eating patterns, children are more likely to follow.

Infants and young children easily show cold symptoms when becoming chilled during sleep. In cold weather, cotton flannel pajamas will keep the child warm. Parents who sleep with their children will know when their children require more insulation from the cold. Family togetherness will also provide extra warmth, love, comfort and protection, so important on cold nights.

Head congestion is an uncomfortable sign of a cold. Many parents buy prepared nose drops and decongestants to help their child feel better. Yet decongestants should not be administered for a runny nose and stuffed head simply because the congestion is the body's only way to drain mucus from the sinuses. One way to begin to relieve the irritated and swollen mucous membranes and to begin draining the sinuses is to use a humidifier or steam to open up clogged air passages.

When my son began eating significant amounts of fruits and vegetables, and drinking green juices, we no longer had to be concerned about ear infections or any other kinds of infections, as the whole picture of illness vanished dramatically in approximately 11 months from the time we began a lifestyle of fresh plant nutrition.

Katrina Blair, founder of Turtle Lake Refuge of Durango, Colorado, and teacher of sustainable living practices and wild edible plant classes, shares some suggestions for sore throat and colds, cold sores and systemic issues such as measles:

"For sore throat, warm lemon water works well as it immediately starts to pull out the congestion and mucus that is creating it. For cold sores, an amino acid called lysine is effective and can be taken orally. Any green juice will be very helpful for shifting the acidity of the body back to an alkaline state of healing."

Plantain is a wonderful wild edible that soothes and heals membranes. Plantain is commonly found in backyards and along roadsides, but be sure to pick it in unsprayed areas.

Eating real organically grown and wild foods is most often the best healer. Dandelion, also a wild edible, is a very nutritious leafy green, loaded with vitamins A, C and K, iron and calcium. It is known to eliminate infections, create bone strength and assist in nerve function. Dandelion helps with digestion and decreases swelling. Many children are not used to eating bitter greens such as dandelion, but we can serve them in ways that allow them to be more easily enjoyed. I make a delicious Dandelion Apple Sauce by blending dandelion leaves with three to four apples and a little water to get it moving in the blender.

All fruits and vegetables, especially if darkly colored, are immune system enhancers, but wild edible plants, such as dandelion, purslane, lambsquarters, sorrel, and wild berries, are among the strongest immune system boosters. Miner's lettuce, another of a powerful wild edible, is rich in vitamins A and C, and is good for eliminating stomach upsets.

Our absolute family favorite natural remedy has always been the warm water bottle. Whether to soothe a stomachache, headache or joint pain, the warm water bottle was our first choice remedy, and we have two or three of them available whenever needed.

▲ ▼ ▲

The Parent Detox

Parents, often overwhelmed with exceptionally full lives, ask about ways to stay healthy with abundant energy, especially when feeling their reserves are being depleted.

When digesting heavier fat and protein foods, we put great stress on the liver and kidneys. What are the foods that cause digestive distress and rob us of our energy? Meat, all animal products, processed and refined carbohydrates as well as eating mainly cooked foods. Parents want to learn how to cleanse from their daily stresses and dysfunctional lifestyle habits. Taking part in a juice or smoothie detoxification, or an even deeper water fast, can be helpful, but I've seen these people return to the same stressful lifestyle and indigestible foods upon completion of their cleanse, until they feel sick and rundown once again.

In addition to the raw food lifestyle of fresh fruits, green leaves, sprouts and vegetables, including smaller amounts of nuts and seeds, which is naturally detoxifying, a weekly one-day water fast is beneficial to keep digestion running smoothly. When water fasting, we give our digestive system a much needed break. Especially when dealing with busy daily schedules, the break

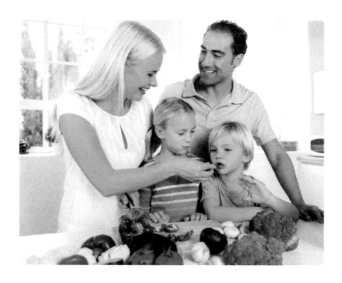

essary and essential water content, so much a part of the cleansing effect of fresh plant foods.

The most beneficial technique for detoxing is eating early in the day, while avoiding eating at night. Whoever has practiced this powerful rejuvenation and health technique cannot stop extolling its virtues:

- Digestion is strongest when the sun is highest.
- Deep, sound sleep is essential to good health.
- When we eat at night, we force the digestion of this food to happen during sleep, thereby diminishing the sleep's focus on cleansing and healing.
- The energy gained through eating in the morning and early afternoon can be used productively throughout the day, but when eating at night, the energy is not used for physical activity and accumulates as fat during sleep.
- We can eliminate waste better in the morning when not eating the night before.
- The rejuvenation and healing benefits of daylight eating are amazing and must be experienced to be believed.

from food for a day each week is extremely healing. For those who prefer to cleanse using food, a green smoothie detox can be life changing. A mix of green leafy vegetables and fruit (for adults I recommend a 60/40 ratio, is made in the blender until smooth, giving the digestive system relief from the constant onslaught of solid foods.

For those living healthfully on fresh raw plant foods, it's important to know that the human system is self-cleaning on these pure fiber-rich foods, as long as one understands the simplicity of the lifestyle. Those who regularly engage in high amounts of nuts and seeds and dehydrated foods will be robbing themselves of the nec-

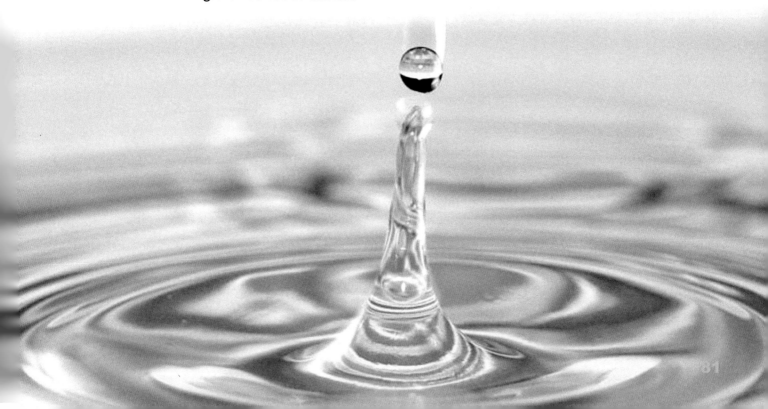

All about Nuts

Q#1: Are raw, organic nuts truly superior to roasted nuts?

A: Raw, organic nuts are definitely superior to roasted nuts. Nuts are sensitive to heat, light and oxygen, the main reasons it's advisable to store nuts and seeds in the freezer to keep them from going rancid. Heat turns their oils rancid, rendering them harmful. When nuts are exposed to the extreme heat of roasting, they are no longer healthful to eat. It makes sense that nuts will always be more healthful in their natural state.

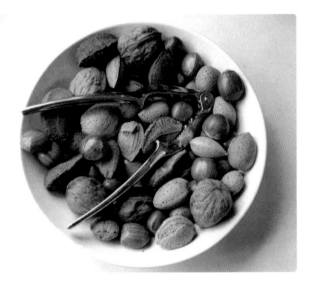

Scientists have tested for the harmful levels of acrylamide, a potentially threatening byproduct of the amino acid asparagine, in roasted nuts such as almonds and hazelnuts. The research results showed that those nuts containing high levels of asparagine released the cancerous chemical compound more than those lacking this amino acid. Nuts rich in asparagine, such as almonds, have the potential to harm your health and fitness when roasted. Opting for raw nuts remains the safest method to avoid such problems. [1] It's difficult today to get truly raw almonds in the United States because there are pasteurization laws in California, where most almonds are grown. However, raw almonds from other areas, such as Sicily, are imported.

Roasting nuts at temperatures higher than 170° Fahrenheit. will cause a breakdown of their fats and the production of free radicals. When nuts roasted commercially at high temperatures are consumed, the free radicals they contain can cause lipid peroxidation—the oxidizing of fats in your bloodstream that can trigger tiny injuries in arterial walls—a first step in the buildup of plaque and cardiovascular disease.[2] Heat has the ability to cause changes in chemical bonds which may affect structures such as fats. High heat can also increase the formation of free radicals, which have negative effects on the body by damaging DNA, the genetic material. These free radicals can also cause a reaction called lipid peroxidation, which can injure blood vessel walls, increasing the risk of heart disease.[3]

Q#2: Why are nut allergies common, and how could a parent avoid this happening to his or her child?

A: An estimated 1.8 million Americans have allergies to tree nuts. Allergic reactions to tree nuts are among the leading causes of fatal and near-fatal reactions to foods. Tree nuts include, but are not limited to, walnuts, almonds, hazelnuts, cashews, pistachios, and Brazil nuts. [4]